Bringing Our Histories into School-Based Therapy

This is a book that delves into the relationship between therapists' sometimes fraught engagement with their own emotional histories and those of their clients, offering a creative template for opening up important conversations.

Each of the chapter authors contributing to this volume focuses on seminal life events that inflect the emotional tenor and quality of attunement in the consulting room. A broad range of subjects is covered, which either highlight themes around identity or reflect the kinds of challenges that bring young people to therapy, including bereavement, the experience of otherness, dislocation and migration, disrupted family relationships, and life-threatening illness.

With compelling clinical vignettes illuminating the resonances between therapists' stories and those of the clients they present, this book is an engaging and insightful read for all practitioners in the field, especially those working in child and adolescent mental health.

Lyn French is a psychotherapist, supervisor, and author with over 25 years' experience in the field of school-based psychotherapy. She is the director of A Space, a psychotherapy service running in partnership with the London Borough of Hackney. A Space and the Institute of International Visual Arts (iniva) have co-published numerous sets of emotional learning cards which use contemporary art along with commentary and questions by Lyn designed to open up conversations in and outside of therapy sessions.

Reva Klein is a child and adolescent counsellor and adult psychoanalytic psychotherapist. She supervises therapists at A Space, and sees clients and supervisees in private practice. Reva has written extensively on children's mental health issues.

"Emotional health comes with a roomy ability to bear a range of feeling states, to 'fold into' our being aspects of ourselves we might otherwise disown. This book is an important contribution to the field of child and adolescent psychotherapy, enabling therapeutic professionals to own our own 'shadows' in the interests of those we work with".

Graham Music, *psychotherapist, trainer, supervisor, lecturer and author*

"Understanding how psychodynamic therapy or counselling works is a challenge for many young people seeking help. This book demonstrates how, after their training, psychotherapists and counsellors are able to use their humanity and life experiences to enable them to provide sensitive, thoughtful help to their young clients whilst retaining a professional boundary. Each author reflects on how young people's stories can resonate with life experiences of their own, leading to a compassionate understanding of the issues adolescents bring to therapy".

Judith Trowell, *consultant child and adolescent psychiatrist, psychoanalyst, child analyst and author*

"What is most distinctive about this rich and enlivening book is the readiness of its writers not only to hold in mind the relevance of their clients' personal histories to their everyday troubled lives, but to reflect on their own backstories and the influence of those experiences on their psychotherapeutic work. They discuss what they themselves bring to the psychotherapeutic relationship - memories, tensions, anxieties - that are not so dissimilar to those of the young people they endeavour to help and which have the power to facilitate or indeed inhibit the therapeutic process. Their self-awareness, which they demonstrate throughout these chapters through vivid narratives, is crucial both to deepen the understanding of young people's problems and to ensure their own appropriate therapeutic discipline in the inevitable intimacy of their psychotherapeutic relationships. It is of great credit to the co-editors and the writers in this book that their explorations of thought and practice are expressed with such refreshing candor as well as courage".

Peter Wilson, *consultant child psychotherapist and founder/ former director of YoungMinds*

"None of us got into this work without reference to our own personal backstories. When it comes to working with children and young people, our own childhoods are especially poignant. While we're all familiar with the idea of 'the wounded healer' in theory, the way in which we integrate our own personal wounds and triumphs into therapy work has been less accessible - until now.

This important book highlights the very human personal journeys and their role in the work we do with children and young people and is a must read for anyone who wants to bring themselves fully, responsibly, and ethically to the work".

Aaron Balick, *psychotherapist, supervisor, author, and director of Stillpoint, an international psychology hub*

Bringing Our Histories into School-Based Therapy

How Therapists' Backstories Enrich
Work with Children and Young People

Edited by
Lyn French and Reva Klein

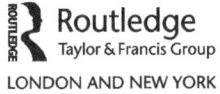

Routledge
Taylor & Francis Group

LONDON AND NEW YORK

Designed cover image: Neeta Madahar *Falling 2* (2005).
Courtesy of the artist and the Institute of International Visual
Arts (iniva) who commissioned the work jointly with Fabrica &
Photoworks. **www.iniva.org**

First published 2023
by Routledge
4 Park Square, Milton Park, Abingdon, Oxon OX14 4RN

and by Routledge
605 Third Avenue, New York, NY 10158

Routledge is an imprint of the Taylor & Francis Group, an informa business

British Library Cataloguing-in-Publication Data
A catalogue record for this book is available from the British Library

Library of Congress Cataloging-in-Publication Data
Names: French, Lyn, 1958– editor. | Klein, Reva, 1951– editor.
Title: Bringing our histories into school-based therapy : how
therapists' backstories enrich work with children and young
people / edited by Lyn French and Reva Klein.
Description: Abingdon, Oxon ; New York, NY : Routledge, 2023. |
Includes bibliographical references and index. |
Identifiers: LCCN 2022053869 (print) | LCCN 2022053870 (ebook) |
ISBN 9781032218892 (hardback) | ISBN 9781032218885 (paperback) |
ISBN 9781003270447 (ebook)
Subjects: LCSH: Child psychotherapy—Great Britain. |
Adolescent psychotherapy—Great Britain. | Counseling in
elementary education—Great Britain. | Counseling in secondary
education—Great Britain. | Psychotherapist and patient—Great
Britain. | Psychotherapists—Mental health—Great Britain. |
Psychotherapists—Great Britain—Attitudes.
Classification: LCC RJ504 .B745 2023 (print) | LCC RJ504 (ebook) |
DDC 618.92/891400941—dc23/eng/20230210
LC record available at https://lccn.loc.gov/2022053869
LC ebook record available at https://lccn.loc.gov/2022053870

ISBN: 9781032218892 (hbk)
ISBN: 9781032218885 (pbk)
ISBN: 9781003270447 (ebk)

DOI: 10.4324/9781003270447

Typeset in Garamond
by codeMantra

For the children and young people with whom we've worked who, without exception, have shown fortitude and commitment in undertaking therapy with us.

Contents

Acknowledgements

We are indebted to A Space for Creative Learning and Support for providing the context for this book. A Space has expanded significantly since its inception in 1997, offering therapeutic services and specialist projects to primary and secondary schools across East London.

We would also like to thank all the past and present trainee and qualified therapists who have brought enthusiasm, dedication, and a drive to learn more to their roles. In addition, we want to acknowledge the many teachers and school staff who have welcomed and supported therapists working with their pupils.

Numerous individuals have made publishing this book possible. In particular, we would like to acknowledge the significant contributions of Alex Sainsbury of the Glass-House Trust (a Sainsbury Family Charitable Trust), Elinor Jansz, Trustee, and Nicola Baboneau, the Chair of A Space.

Routledge editors Joanne Forshaw, Grace McDonnell, and Georgina Clutterbuck provided steady support and guidance throughout, for which we warmly thank them.

Contributors

Marta Alonso completed her Psychology BSC in Spain with a specialism in Neuropsychology and moved to the UK to take up the opportunity to develop a wider approach to her practice. Having always been part of theatre, dance, and visual arts projects she shifted her focus to exploring the role of the arts in an evidence-based approach to psychotherapy. On completing her Art Psychotherapy post-graduate training and working as a therapist in educational settings for over a decade Marta developed a puppetry-based model of group therapy with the aim of reaching a wider number of children in need of emotional support. She continues to deliver puppetry-based psycho-educational and therapeutic programmes in schools and mental health provisions. Marta also works for A Space providing longer-term individual therapy in mainstream and special needs secondary school.

Mihoko Arayama is a psychodynamic counsellor and psychotherapist. She originally qualified as a clinical psychologist in Japan where she gained rich experiences of working with children with learning disabilities and other special needs including autism and very low birth weight. She conducted assessments and took part in therapeutic groups where she increased her level of understanding of mother–infant interactions. She also worked extensively with school refusal both in groups and with individuals when the issue first became a phenomenon in Japan. Determined to pursue her interest in mother–infant relationships and to engage in further professional training, Mihoko moved to the UK. Following her post-graduate training at the Tavistock, she completed the psychodynamic counselling and psychotherapy with children and adolescents MSc at Birkbeck College, University of London. She currently works for A Space providing services in secondary school settings and has a private practice offering individual therapy as well as supervision.

Farah Bajull is a psychodynamic art therapist whose primary interest is in the use of art as an expressive and exploratory tool. She has worked with children, adolescents, and adults spanning a wide range of cultural backgrounds. She also pioneered the use of art psychotherapy for older people in an institution that provides dementia respite and end-of-life care. Together, these roles have given her insights into the development of individuals from infancy to old age, along with an understanding of specific life-cycle challenges. She currently works for A Space providing services in secondary school settings, as well as maintaining a private practice alongside her artistic practice. As a graduate of Chelsea College of Arts and the Royal College of Arts, she has exhibited internationally including 'Veil', organised by iniva (Institute of International Visual Arts) in collaboration with Modern Art Oxford. Through her artistic and psychotherapy practice, she aims to share the creative process with others, connecting them with their innate creativity and enhancing their wellbeing.

Margery Craig is a child and adolescent psychotherapist and adult psychoanalytic psychotherapist. Margery's first experience in this field was during her career as a designer when she began to volunteer in her spare time on a national helpline for children. After many years of speaking to young people as a volunteer, the charity offered her a role as a counselling supervisor and trainer, prompting a change in her career direction. At the same time she embarked on the Birkbeck MSc in Psychodynamic Counselling for Children and Adolescents in order to broaden her knowledge and skills. On graduating Margery combined her established role at the national children's charity with work at A Space, where she offered services to both primary and secondary age children. Over time Margery's interest led her to undertake a second clinical training at the Guild of Psychotherapists and as she moved forward, alongside her role as a lead therapist in an academy working with students and staff, she was seeing adults in an NHS Specialist Psychotherapy Service and in a third sector clinic. Margery now works as a psychotherapist in private practice seeing adults and adolescents.

Angie Doran is a counsellor working in Sixth Form colleges for A Space and a psychotherapist in private practice. She completed an MSc in psychodynamic counselling and psychotherapy with children and adolescents at Birkbeck College, University of London, before taking the role of lead researcher on a joint PhD project set up by A Space with the Centre for Psychoanalytic Studies at the University of Essex. Some of the findings from this study were published by Angie in the article 'Informed Outcomes: Self-rating measures and their use in psychodynamic therapy with adolescents', in the *Journal of Psychodynamic Practice* 19(1) and in *Therapeutic Practice in Schools Vol II: The Contemporary Adolescent* co-edited by Lyn French and Reva Klein. She also contributed to the first volume, both published by Routledge. In her work at A Space spanning a 13-year period, Angie has been responsible for setting up services in primary and secondary schools, as well as in Sixth Form colleges. She has also had a lead role in establishing psychotherapy, supervision, and consultation for school staff as part of the A Space provision.

Josephine Evans trained on the MSc Course as a child and adolescent psychotherapist at Birkbeck College, University of London. During her time at A Space as a schools-based counsellor, she was responsible for setting up new counselling services in primary and secondary schools, developing Year 6/7 transition support projects, seeing school staff for counselling and supervising university student trainees on placement. In addition, Jo was involved in workshops and presentations jointly led by A Space and the Institute of International Visual Arts (iniva) contributing to research on the use of contemporary art as a starting point for psycho-social development. Jo has also been a regular guest lecturer at Birkbeck University, delivering seminars on working as a counsellor in schools, and more specifically working with adolescents. Over the years bereavement has become her specialism about which she has written (*Therapeutic Practice in Schools Vol II: The Contemporary Adolescent*). Jo worked previously in the arts for 20 years as an actor/musician, performing at the National Theatre and in the West End, touring and repertory theatre, film and television. She currently runs a service as an independent counsellor at a secondary school in South London. More recently, Jo has instigated links between the school she is based in and the South London Gallery to develop arts-based school and community projects and resources to address and raise awareness of systemic racism and structural inequalities, particularly within education.

Lyn French is an art therapist and psychoanalytic psychotherapist. She was one of the original team members contracted in 1997 to set up 'A Space for creative learning & support', a partnership between Alex Sainsbury of the Glass-House Trust (a Sainsbury Family Charitable Trusts), the Social Science Research Unit (Institute of Education, University of London), and Hackney Education. She has been the director since 2000 and continues to oversee service delivery across schools in East London as well as taking a lead role in any research undertaken. A partnership established in the early 2000s between A Space and the Institute of International Visual Arts (iniva) has resulted in many artist and therapist-led initiatives. Out of this work, Lyn co-developed sets of emotional learning cards with iniva featuring contemporary art and psychologically resonant commentary and questions which are sold internationally through iniva's website. Along with Reva Klein, Lyn co-edited *Therapeutic Practice in Schools: Working with the Child Within* and *Therapeutic Practice in Schools Volume 2: The Contemporary Adolescent* both published by Routledge. For over ten years, she was a sessional lecturer on the MSc in psychodynamic counselling and psychotherapy with children and adolescents at Birkbeck College, University of London.

Angela Ike After a degree in Journalism and Psychology, Angela worked as a writer before retraining as a psychodynamic counsellor and then completing a master's in Psychotherapeutic Counselling. As a counsellor, she has worked in various organisations including a service for male survivors of sexual violence, a secondary school, and an online counselling service for young people. Angela has worked in higher education for several years and is currently senior counsellor with the counselling service at the University of Cambridge. She has a special interest in transgenerational trauma, social constructionism, and the impact these factors can have on an individual's inner world and sense of self. Angela has some experience of teaching on a Psychodynamic Counselling course at the Centre for Psychoanalytic Studies at the University of Essex and is currently a supervisor in training. Her master's dissertation was entitled *What are the experiences of Afro Caribbean trainee Counsellors and Psychotherapists with regards to the notions of race being addressed or otherwise within their clinical supervision?* It is available on the BAATN website.

Sue Kegerreis is professor at the Department of Psychosocial and Psychoanalytic Studies at the University of Essex, where she set up and runs the MA in Psychodynamic Counselling. She formerly established the MSc in Psychodynamic Counselling with Children and Adolescents at Birkbeck. Trained first at the Tavistock and then at the Lincoln, she has worked with children, adolescents and adults in CAMHS and in hospital and school settings as well as privately. She has taught on a wide range of courses and published widely on clinical and training issues. She is particularly engaged with promoting research among psychodynamic practitioners and recently re-launched the Professional Doctorate for counsellors and psychotherapists at the University of Essex. She is managing editor of *Psychodynamic Practice.*

Reva Klein is a child and adolescent counsellor and adult psychoanalytic psychotherapist who supervises therapists at A Space and sees clients and supervisees in private practice. Previously a freelance journalist, writer, and editor, Reva taught journalism at Goldsmiths College for many years. She is the author of three books on education – *Defying Disaffection, Citizens by Right,* and *We Want our Say* – and is the co-author of *Reluctant Refuge: The Story of Asylum in Britain.* She twice won the Commission for Racial Equality's Race in the Media Award for her writing in the Times Educational Supplement, and she founded and edited *The International Journal on School Disaffection,* an Anglo-American publication now in its second decade. In the 1990s Reva sat on the Secondary School Reform Committee of UNESCO. Along with Lyn French, Reva co-edited *Therapeutic Practice in Schools: Working with the Child Within* and *Therapeutic Practice in Schools: The Contemporary Adolescent* both published by Routledge.

Melanie Light started as an advertising copywriter, learning the art of succinct communication. After having children, she moved into education and soon became interested in the 'unsuccinct' communication behind behaviour and the emotional blocks to learning. She consequently enrolled on the MSc Course in Child and Adolescent Counselling and Psychotherapy at Birkbeck

College, University of London. She is now based in primary and secondary schools as a counsellor, working with students and school staff, and as a supervisor at A Space for Creative Learning and Support in the London Borough of Hackney.

Tony McLeod is a psychoanalytically informed behavioural specialist. He has worked in many different schools and settings with a range of pupils whose behaviour was a clear communication of a troubling and troubled inner world. His interest in the psychological and emotional impact of children who are taken into care has grown since he and his partner adopted two boys. This led to training in therapeutic parenting which promotes using attachment and trauma-informed relational skills and strategies also of relevance to teachers, teaching assistants, and therapists working with neurodiverse children and young people. Along with other parents, Tony was instrumental in forming We are Family (WAF), now a fully established charity in its own right and an invaluable support for adopters and prospective adopters. Following a period away from work on parental leave, Tony is now taking up a new position providing therapeutic support in an alternative educational provision in north London.

Martina Nalesso has a background in Fine Arts and gained a master's degree in Art Education from the Academy of Fine Arts in Venice, Italy before qualifying as an art psychotherapist at the University of Roehampton in London (UK). She has experience of working with children as an art facilitator in community events and museums, and of delivering art workshops with adults suffering from mental health issues. Following her art psychotherapy training, she has focused on school-based practice and has amassed considerable experience of working with children and young people with autism and complex learning difficulties. She currently works in primary and secondary schools and Sixth Form colleges both with A Space in Hackney and independently in a secondary school in a neighbouring borough. She continues to stay in touch with her creative side and uses art to express herself mainly through painting, photography, collage, and embroidery.

Stefania Putzu-Williams completed her first degree in Psychology at Rome University before receiving an MA in Psychoanalytic Observational Studies at the Tavistock Clinic/UCL and an MSc in Psychodynamic Counselling at Birkbeck. She is also a chartered psychologist in Italy. After writing a thesis on child abuse in the UK, she began specialising in the care of children and young people and has worked therapeutically since 1989. From in-depth experience including residential assessment of high-risk families prior to Family Court decisions, she has developed expertise as a counsellor in community and school-based projects (for over ten years within CAMHS), and in more recent years, as a counsellor at Bacon's College in Southwark. She also works as a clinical supervisor in private practice.

Gwendolyn Rowlands is an art psychotherapist who works with children and adolescents in schools. After training as a sculptor, she established a studio practice and exhibiting career. In tandem with this she worked in Further Education for 17 years as a sculpture tutor offering non-vocational studio-based courses to adult learners. The experience of teaching adults to develop their creativity and self-expression opened up questions regarding the therapeutic possibilities of art-making in support of good mental health. She pursued this interest by volunteering for a number of years for a national mental health charity. Initially concerned with adult mental health Gwendolyn became interested in child development during her art psychotherapy MA at Roehampton University. Since then, she has continued to specialise in this area working with children from five years old through to young people in Sixth Form with A Space and Place2Be. As an art psychotherapist Gwendolyn maintains a daily drawing practice. As well as offering a way of linking with clients and their expressions it allows her a space to sustain her own wellbeing.

David Trevatt was born in London and grew up in Liverpool in the 1950s and 1960s. He moved back to London in the 1970s graduating in Social Sciences and then qualifying as a social worker. He worked in many different settings in social work including attachment to schools, and attended various training programmes, mainly at the Tavistock Clinic, where he eventually undertook Child Psychotherapy training. Since qualification he worked in several Child and Adolescent Services (CAMHS), both in NHS teams and the voluntary sector. He developed interests in consultation with parents and organisations in private practice, research, teaching, and supervision. He retired in 2014 and lives on the Isle of Wight.

Foreword

Graham Music

It is with great pleasure that I write the foreword to this book. The subject matter is dear to my heart and the issues are too little discussed or written about. Each of us who works with children, whether in schools or elsewhere, has, of course, our own very particular life experiences as children, as pupils, as peers, and these all inevitably inform how we approach the work we do. We know the extent to which school years are extremely formative ones for brains, bodies, nervous systems, psyches, the development of memories, social capacities, and so much more, albeit differently so at primary age and in adolescence. Such memories are often visceral, and we know now how emotions are felt in the body. I still feel a wave of anxiety that belongs to my teenage self when I go into a big secondary school to give a talk, or a sinking feeling when I smell something that reminds me of the boiled cabbage odour at a school where I was bullied. We must process our own experiences if we are to do this work well, and this in turn can help us reach out to the children we see.

I have long been a passionate advocate of taking therapeutic services into school. Over the years, I have set up about 50 services, and these have helped thousands of young people as well as families, teachers and SEN staff. It is one of my proudest achievements. A new adolescent therapy service in East London, Hear and Now, soon had therapists in every single secondary school. At the Tavistock Clinic I set up TOPS (Tavistock Outreach Project in Schools) which worked with a range of primary schools for over 20 years. A few years later, I also set up a service in a partnership between the Tavistock and Camden Primary Care Trust (PCT) placing an experienced therapist into every mainstream and specialist secondary school in the Borough for two days a week. What was always fascinating in supervising such work was the unique chemical reactions between each school's specific culture, history, and ways of treating children and the particular personality traits, skills, and personal histories of each therapist. We might think that in good therapeutic work the therapist, but also the school, becomes what Bollas (1989) described as a transformational object allowing a young person's potential self to be realised.

My own history has greatly influenced my approach, including which children I was best able to work with myself and most suited to help teachers and therapists understand. I was an anxious kid myself who had many embarrassing and unsavoury habits which were mainly in the service of closing down feelings I could not manage. As described in a recent book, *Respark* (Music, 2022), my habits included sucking on my school tie so that it developed a nasty texture and an unrecognisable shape. Others included jiggling my legs when others hoped I would sit still, or being disruptive when my hypervigilant self felt triggered, and/or when I did not get the exercise my hyperactive symptoms needed. I also was highly, or hyper, sensitive, flinching at loud sounds, and anticipating danger around every corner. For me, powerful feelings were difficult to manage, and I needed to defend against them, but needless to say, they often got me into trouble.

Once I hit adolescence, I escaped from hormone-induced overwhelm by reading a book a day, the more complex and philosophical the better. While this opened my mind and vistas, it also stopped me feeling feelings I could not manage. My own adolescent experience enabled me to work with and not be taken in by the bright, jumpy, and sometimes dazzling minds of some of my clients, and instead to reach for the softer, more desperate feelings below the surface with a degree of compassion that I first needed to show myself. This meant finding some kind of third space – not stuck in our own preoccupations, nor that of the young person.

Sometimes of course we get too stuck in our own issues, overidentified with a child, or parent, or teacher. For example, I am generally quite good at loss and mourning, having worked through much of my own. But I recall one child I initially failed, whose mother was dying at the time that I was undergoing a bereavement of my own and who I thought was more ready than they were to face an unthinkable impending loss. We did recover in that case, but therapeutic failures are so often linked to a therapist's blind-spots and inability to process countertransference dynamics.

Schools of course can often judge a child for their behaviour, becoming critical, exasperated, angry, and indeed, punitive, something I have long written about (Music, 2008) and know well personally. I knew first hand as an unhappy child how easy it was to be told off for acting out when anxious or depressed, or to be ignored or thought odd or strange when I was going through emotional agony, or depression, or low confidence.

It is all too easy to perceive defences against emotional pain as a problem, as behaviours to change, when in fact they are ways of contracting in the face of anxiety, an attempt to push away feelings that are too much to bear. Such defences give rise to a tightening in our muscles and in our very beings, a wariness of others, a lack of trust, and a closing down of hope. When in adolescence I buried my head in books I was defending against overwhelming feelings, but also developing a contracted attitude to life. This left me, as it does many adolescents, feeling very alone.

Emotional health comes with a roomy ability to bear a range of feeling states, to 'fold in' to our being aspects of ourselves we might otherwise disown. As an adolescent I had to deny and hide from myself and others much that I felt, like insecurity, vulnerability, jealousy, or hurt. It is hard to explain the palpable relief on the few occasions when this was noticed, when one teacher saw I had 'sad eyes', which I did not know, and another realised that my shrinking handwriting was a sign of an emotional issue. I did not realise these things about myself, but when empathised with and understood, it allowed my whole being to relax and literally to breathe more easily.

When I started out organising therapeutic services, I did not much understand trauma, but I knew emotionally of its effects. I too was bullied at primary school, and remember all too well the fear and terror when a tough local kid picked on me. I was threatened, and tried to hide wherever I could in the toilets, the classroom, a shed, anywhere. On one occasion when a teacher ordered me to go out into the playground, I knew what was coming. The bully sauntered up to me snarling and scowling, shouted my name, his fist raised. In that moment I felt terrified, my legs becoming jelly, I was rooted to the spot, barely breathing, my stomach knotted, knowing I had nowhere to flee. As he started to hit me, I tried to fight back. I had never fought anyone and sadly, this story did not have a good ending, as I was kicked and hit and, in my memory, surrounded by taunting kids. The next time it happened there was no muscular tension, I went floppy, faint, felt sick. I became insular, inward, and could not tell anyone.

This went on for weeks, and I remember the feeling of going cold, immobilising, and on several occasions, almost watching myself from outside my body as I was being punched. Luckily after some time the bully left the school. Also I could redeem myself, mainly as I was good at sports which allowed me a modicum of acceptance, even popularity. However, I had regular nightmares and inside felt ashamed and terrified. Something of the numbness and bad memories remained for many years. It was only my own therapy, decades later, that brought me back to myself. I of course needed that help then, and that is just what school therapists, such as this book's contributors, can offer, and nowadays they can do this with an understanding of trauma which was lacking not so long ago.

Without such help I could not think about my experiences, and in turn I could not help the children and families I was working with or therapists I was supervising. In trauma people can literally become 'thoughtless', go into a stupor (stupefaction), and become speechless. It leaves people feeling unsafe to the core of their beings. It was because I knew this so deeply in myself that I tried to prioritise the children who were silently struggling and were easy to miss.

My personal history includes being sent away to school at the age of nine, where I, alongside others my age, had to just 'get on with it', where there was no space for moping, missing parental care, or expecting emotional understanding or support. Many of us developed tough defences, exoskeletons, which helped our survival, but left our needy, vulnerable selves unseen and deeply buried. The boys who cried at night were often teased for being weak and sissies. We needed to hide our pain and despair. The psychoanalyst Herbert Rosenfield

(1987) described how needy, dependent parts of the self can be disowned and denigrated, resulting in a hatred of vulnerability, in ourselves and others. We responded like this to the crying boys, from whom we were determined to differentiate ourselves. I often feel like crying now for the boys whose pain was not recognised and who so badly needed understanding.

It is so easy to miss children with cut-off presentations, including the very shy ones, and I was one of those too. Teachers and pastoral support staff often get frustrated with them. When in the company of people who are emotionally cut-off, we can experience feelings like boredom, frustration, or lack of interest. Such feelings are hard and even embarrassing to admit to for therapists who like to be thought of as warm, empathic, and kind. Yet humans are a resonant species and with people in avoidant states of mind we can find ourselves feeling dulled down, thoughts becoming wooden and bodily feelings, flat. I think such resonating gives us a hint of what it must be like to live in their skin.

Staying emotionally open to the other can be the toughest task, especially when we see them as different, bad, naughty, lazy, as not trying. These are all labels that can be used when distancing from another and making them other. Several of the chapters in this book sensitively describe issues of sameness and difference, of identity and being an outsider. In our world today we have to be more aware than ever of issues of identity, in particular around race and ethnicity as well as culture, gender, and sexuality. It is as easy for us as therapists to show unconscious bias as it is for anyone else; in fact we all inevitably do. Our non-conscious expectations mean we often see what is not there, whether it's the anxious black face as threatening or the scared child as aggressive, just as the traumatised or fearful adolescent might see disapproval or disdain where none is there.

'Othering', whether in racial bias or dehumanision, or disowning parts of ourselves, goes against what we as therapists should be doing if we are to truly help the children who come into our care. We need to reach out to parts of ourselves we would rather disown, as only then can we reach out to the other, especially the aspects of a child or young person that can trigger us. The best help is always served up in compassionate, safe human relationships with a curious and empathic other who can enjoy us, bear pain and despair with us, and show that there is more to life than what our numbed body/mind/heart believes. Personally I did not have enough of this when young, but I had a few experiences which stayed with me illustrating just how much it means when someone can see past the defensive façade or 'bad behaviours' to the struggling person inside. All children need a compassionate other to reach out to them, whether a parent or caregiver, or another adult, professional, therapist, friend, or mentor. We all need someone to turn to when we are in trouble, something I know in myself and see week-in-week-out with nearly all my clients.

As someone who has rarely felt they have belonged, which is partly explained by both my individual and ethnic history, I know how easy it is to not feel genuinely met and seen, nor to really meet the other for who they are, as Buber (2002) and Levinas et al. (1996) both exhorted us to aspire to. Identity and difference are and should be a central preoccupation for everyone in today's world, and of course for therapists. But staying open and interested and not judging the other is a tall order. I have found this particularly in work with, for example, perpetrators of violence or sexual offences. Remembering the victim in the perpetrator and trying to understand them, as well as staring 'evil in the eye' and also owning the perpetrator aspects of ourselves, opens the possibility of integration and reduces the risks of splitting and projection. This requires deep psychic work, honesty, and the courage to stay with what we would rather deny or push away.

This book is an important contribution to such a project and helps to enable the therapeutic professions to own our own 'shadows' in the interests of those we work with. Many in the psychoanalytic world might not approve of such self-disclosure. But I think the relational tradition (e.g., Aron, 2001) has taught us about the myths of neutrality and a genuine blank screen as well as the dangers of being both too emotionally neutral and too drawn into transference–countertransference dynamics.

With luck, and help, we can all internalise loving, compassionate care in the form of a part of the self which we carry inside us and which we can go to when we are in trouble. Psychoanalysis talks of developing a 'good internal object' and others such as Paul Gilbert describe inner compassionate figures (Gilbert, 2019). I also like the metaphor of another internal figure, what Symington has called the lifegiver (Symington, 1993). It is this lifegiver which, when we feel safe enough, can then help us reach out to hope, joy, and playfulness too – in effect to the good things that life has to offer. I have recently been suggesting that good therapeutic work starts with what I call *safening*, that ability to feel at ease and safe and respected in the presence of another. It is from that position that we have the potential to uncontract and reboot and open up to life's rich possibilities. Being body-aware of our own and others' somatic states, what I have called 'nervous-system whispering', is needed to be able to offer first a safening, then a reset, a reboot, and in time a resparking that generates an embodied lifeforce and energy. This all depends on good human connection with an empathic, compassionate other. To offer this we need to give this to ourselves, and this book contributes to this possibility.

References

Aron, L. 2001. *A meeting of minds: Mutuality in psychoanalysis.* New York: Analytic Press.

Bollas, C. 1989. *Forces of destiny: Psychoanalysis and human idiom.* London: Free Association Books.

Buber, M. 2002. *Between man and man.* London: Routledge.

Gilbert, P. 2019. Explorations into the nature and function of compassion. *Current Opinion in Psychology.* 28, pp. 108–114.

Levinas, E., Peperzak, A.T., Critchley, S. and Bernasconi, R. 1996. *Emmanuel levinas: Basic philosophical writings.* Bloomington, IN: Indiana University Press.

Music, G. 2008. From scapegoating to thinking and finding a home: Delivering thera-peutic work in schools. *Journal of Child Psychotherapy*. 34(1), pp. 43–61.

Music, G. 2022. *RESPARK: Igniting hope and joy after trauma and depression*. London: Mind-Nurturing Books.

Rosenfeld, H.A. 1987. *Impasse and interpretation: Therapeutic and anti-therapeutic factors in the psycho-analytic treatment of psychotic, borderline, and neurotic patients*. Oxford: Routledge.

Symington, N. 1993. *Narcissism: A new theory*. London: Karnac Books.

Introduction

Lyn French and Reva Klein

In the early 2000s, one of the first 'Teach-ins' hosted by the newly formed *Relational School UK* was held in a large lecture theatre in a university in Central London, hired for the day. Following the usual programme for such events, it began with the presentation of papers. However, no one stuck to the script. Each speaker brought in pivotal moments in their own personal history relating to the themes they were discussing. The result was electric, bringing the morning alive in a way that most of us hadn't experienced before. This wasn't done gratuitously or simply for effect. Central to relational psychotherapy is the idea that our own life experiences affect the tone and tenor of our presence in the consulting room fuelling a deep interest in enactments, intersubjectivity and transference–countertransference dynamics. Our early life, as well as those seminal moments, shape who we are which, in turn, influences our choice of theory and technique. This is a subject Maroda (2022) thoroughly and illuminatingly unpacks in *The Analyst's Vulnerability* in which she examines what is often unspoken and undisclosed. She notes how "we often favour theoretical approaches and interventions that sometimes fall too easily into either a repetition of our own pasts or a defence against experiencing that repetition." (Ibid, Introduction)

The importance of delving into our innermost self and making the unconscious conscious is reflected in all psychotherapy trainings which have personal analysis as a core requirement. Until more recent years, the idea of bringing some of this material into the public forum was considered a step too far. Adherence to the concept of the analyst's abstinence – the proverbial 'blank screen' – meant that even within our professional community, self-disclosure was rare. In the introduction to *Clinical Implications of the Psychoanalyst's Life Experience: When the Personal Becomes Professional* (2014), Steven Kuchuck writes,

> There is, of course, a tremendous irony that our profession's not-too-long ago (and for some, still current) ego ideal was to hide the analyst's true self or certain … self-states – often at great psychological cost for both analyst and patient – as a part of the process of helping patients to come out of hiding and uncover a fuller range of these states.
>
> (2014:20)

DOI: 10.4324/9781003270447-1

It is not uncommon for trainees to privately worry that their fractured, often shame-based, history has left them too flawed to have 'the right' to work in this profession. On the contrary: being in touch with what is usually hidden from view – initially, our own included – is essential if we are to work through it. We think that selective sharing can not only enliven texts but also helpfully lessen the sometimes more extreme asymmetry of the therapist/client dyad. Graham Music's *Respark: Igniting hope and joy after trauma and depression* (2022) is a masterclass in doing just this. He manages to weave in references to his own growing up years which add to his insights while also infusing his writing with humility and humanity.

The origins of this book trace back a decade to the time when we introduced the theme of bringing our histories into our in-house work discussion groups at **A Space for Support**, a school-based therapy service set up in 1997 by Alex Sainsbury (Director, The Glass-house Trust, a Sainsbury Family Charitable Trust) in partnership with the Social Science Research Unit at the Institute of Education, University of London and Hackney Education. Most of the chapters are written by psychotherapists who are currently, or have recently, been members of the A Space team. Those who haven't are known to us via our networks. All have worked in primary/secondary schools, Sixth Form Colleges and universities and/or are supervising therapists based in schools. The majority have presented a paper at A Space drawing on their life experiences which was our starting point. The material brought to these sessions contributed to our thinking about young clients' family stories including the ways in which the histories of previous generations echo down the line, often informing perceptions of self/other relationships.

Each author was invited to either re-work their paper or, for the few who hadn't presented, to start from scratch. Either way, this was no easy task: we were asking them to discuss key experiences in a way that would respect family members who were – and still may be – part of their story while also revealing enough to give emotional texture and depth to their chapter. Moreover, the personal material described was to be linked to themes or life events that bring young people to therapy. As contributing authors ourselves, we know what an emotional and intellectual challenge this was.

A recurring theme in working in the field of child and adolescent psychotherapy is that of identity. As conceptualising and constructing a sense of self is a lifelong task that begins in earnest in early adolescence, a number of chapter authors illustrate how in-depth reflection on our own experiences puts us in touch with key issues and concerns inherent in any exploration of identity. Our premise is that school-based therapists benefit from understanding what can influence this process, something which a number of the personal stories included in this book highlight. With migration set to increase worldwide over coming decades, in part due to the impact of political conflict, war and climate change, themes covered such as insider/outsider-ness; belonging and not belonging; and carrying two or more 'internal worlds' relating to one's birth country and one's adopted home will all be relevant to immigrants or children of migrants.

As each therapist's story is unique, the chapter format has not been standard-ised. The part-fictionalised clinical vignettes, where included, have been created to capture some of the recurring themes in school-based therapy. They illumi-nate the resonances between our stories and those of our clients which serve to illustrate how the tragedies, complexities, and ambiguities of life, as well as les-sons learned, can be thought about from different perspectives. The importance of holding the tension between identifying with aspects of the client's story and ensuring that we do not make assumptions based on our own experiences is emphasised. Even when there is no direct link between our experience and that of our clients, our own sometimes fraught engagement with our emotional histories provides us with a creative template for opening up important conver-sations with children and adolescents.

As our aim is to explore the therapist's subjectivity and to encourage think-ing about how it can influence how we make sense of our clients' stories, we do not discuss or debate the use of self-disclosure as a therapeutic tool. Whether or not, or when, disclosure is used in therapy are complex questions, usually ones which are considered on a case-by-case basis. Instead, through thoughtfully and compassionately illuminating aspects of our own backstories, we demon-strate the value of closely examining one's own personal history in the fullest sense, disentangling the kinds of conscious and unconscious threads which run through every story. At the same time, by revealing some of our struggles, we hope to convey the notion that space can usefully be made in our own minds and within our professional communities for our vulnerabilities, traumas, confusion, and shame to be acknowledged and thought about. Staying in touch with past and present complexities not only keeps us connected to our human fallibilities but greatly enriches our practice. Therapists, like our clients, grapple with test-ing challenges, which is something we need not speak openly about but which nonetheless contributes to the emotional depth of our work with young people.

Building multi-layered and nuanced narratives over time is central to psy-chodynamically informed therapy. So too is facing the attendant anxiety and guilt that can arise, as well as experiencing the pleasure in making connections and the relief in 'seeing and being seen'. Although all of us as contributing au-thors are trained psychodynamically (or in the case of Tony McLeod, use ideas from applied psychoanalysis), this is not the sole approach taken in their school-based therapy. We all incorporate a range of methodologies in the aid of iden-tifying and working on unhelpful core beliefs and unconscious biases. Helping clients to become aware of the stories they tell themselves about themselves and their place in the world, as well as supporting them in modifying self-defeating or overly negative thinking, is key to our work. The capacity to mentalise, that is, to be able to understand the ways in which our mental state and that of oth-ers can influence perception and behaviour, is a core relational skill, one which child and adolescent therapists support young people in developing.

Although the school-based therapist's practice is necessarily pluralistic, the analysis and interpretation that chapter authors apply to their stories and those of their clients demonstrate how we use psychoanalytic thinking when reflecting on the material brought to us. By including careful examination of our own life events, we hope that readers will be encouraged to think about their experiences and the unique ways in which these can affect their clinical understanding, theoretical interests, and transference/countertransference dynamics in their work with children and young people.

Over ten years' experience of using the personal to reflect on the clinical in our A Space work discussion groups has shown us how the key preoccupations of psychoanalysis – loss, mourning, anxiety, guilt, shame, ambivalence, insider/outsider-ness, sense of self, emotional damage inflicted and received, and intergenerational trauma – play out in the construction of the self, our relationships, and our own histories. Mining our own stories with honesty and self-compassion helps us to better understand ourselves and our young clients, spanning the world within and without.

Chapter 1

Not a blank slate

The role of our history in our therapeutic work

Sue Kegerreis

Introduction – the personal story of the therapist

Charlotte (not her real name) tells me about her relationship with her older sister in her first counselling session. The 15-year-old explains how she always looked up to her, even idolised her, wanting above all else to be like her and to be liked by her. She talks about how her mother seems to prefer her sister, lighting up when she was with her while Charlotte always feels just tolerated by her mother, and always worries that she is annoying or boring her. She feels despised by her sister and is confused by the intensity of both hate and hopeless love that she feels.

For me, this is difficult. I am listening to Charlotte, but at the same time am flooded with the familiarity of what is being described. Memories of these dynamics and the feelings that went with them rise unbidden in my mind and I struggle to stay fully connected with Charlotte. She could be my 15-year-old self without much translation.

What happens next, of course, could go in many ways. The identification I feel with Charlotte could lead to my being unable to differentiate between my former self and this young person sitting in the room with me. I could assume I know what she feels and why. I could stop tuning into the utterly unique dilemmas and conflicts that she faces. Crucially, I could miss the way in which her situation is very different from mine. For example, her father is not at all like mine and her parents' relationship is intense and conflicted but loving with a completely different oedipal triangulation in place. Her mother is far more actively involved in the generation of the rivalry, and Charlotte herself is much less competitive and less angry and driven than I was. But if I am overwhelmed by my identification with Charlotte it could be difficult to see these differences. I might be so fired up with the need to rescue her from what is effectively my own pain that I end up leaving her feeling misheard or misunderstood.

Or the opposite could happen. The familiarity of these feelings could lend my interventions just that bit more of an empathic charge, while not interfering with my appreciation of her individuality. I could offer her a sense of being accepted and understood, without missing that she requires just as much

DOI: 10.4324/9781003270447-2

focussed thought to understand as any other young person. I might try just that bit harder, in fact, to tune into her unique emotional dynamics, stimulated by the knowledge that I have struggled myself with some of this but not with exactly what she is wrestling with. She may unconsciously sense my emotional investment in helping her sort out her own feelings in relation to her sister without finding herself acting as a proxy for my own 15-year-old self who so badly wanted someone to listen to her own woes.

Or here is another scenario. Adina, 16, comes to see me and talks about her intense irritation with her younger brother. She can't stand the way he wants to be with her all the time and wishes him gone. She finds his impingements on her infuriating and can't bear it when her brother gets any attention from her parents. She simply cannot understand why they have any time for him at all and recounts with indignation a story of being told off for not being kind to him. It is hard for me to listen to this dispassionately and to make enough space for what this means to this particular young woman. My identification with the younger sibling, even though again there are major differences in the family dynamics, makes it difficult not to take up cudgels on his behalf and to seek to find a way of helping her be more understanding of his feelings. While there might be room for this in the work with her, my capacity to tune in and be empathic with her anxieties and insecurities is in danger of being crowded out with my personal need for the younger sibling to be treated better.

This book is about the role of our own growing up stories in relation to our work, particularly with adolescents. We all know that some adolescents speak to us with particular power, when they tap into the still vividly remembered episodes of our own lives. We remember little of our infancy and often do not have clear recollections of our latency feelings, partly as these are too far in the past for detailed memory, but also because we are so different from our latency selves. We may not fully comprehend why we made some of the decisions we made in adolescence, but we may well remember what it felt like to be facing those dilemmas, and might recall, often with vivid, even excruciating feelings, our adventures and misadventures as teenagers. How often have we woken at three o'clock in the morning with the shame and pain of one of our adolescent mis-steps unbelievably still upsetting us after all this time, and a great deal of therapy, with diminished but still significant power. Maybe that is just me, but I do not think so.

Is this 'countertransference'?

If we use the term countertransference to relate to everything we feel about and experience with clients then it might be thought that this is what is at issue here. However, even in its earliest incarnation this concept was not intended to include the conscious influence of actual memories, but was more connected to unconscious dynamics at work in the relationship. In the first formulations, countertransference referred to the way our own unresolved conflicts, those aspects of our own pasts which we have not fully been able to process emotion-ally, can get tangled up with the therapeutic relationship and interfere with our capacity to operate in a fully professional way with our clients. Freud's original formulation of countertransference as a concept was about this. His approach was strongly influenced by the fact that several of his followers and friends (Breuer, Jung and Ferenczi) were getting into complicated emotional and sexual relationships with their patients, (the latter two having affairs) which Freud saw as these men being swayed by the transference dynamics as a result of not being sufficiently analysed themselves. He advocated (1912) that the analyst should seek further therapy to avoid these pitfalls and to restore their function as a 'mirror' to the patient's projections, primarily in order that the reaction to the analyst could be used to throw light on the patient's own way of relating and their old conflicts.

Ideas about the countertransference have come a very long way since then, (e.g. Heimann 1949, Racker 1948 and Carpy 1989) with it now having a differ-ent set of meanings. In recent times countertransference is seen as being much more about how awareness of the feelings and responses aroused in the thera-pist in the work can be used as a sensitive instrument, finely tuned to pick up nuances of the relational field created by the client. Our own unresolved con-flicts can derail us with our patients for sure, but this is conceptually different from the way in which we are drawn into the relational world of our clients by how they are with us and what their unconscious communications bring to the surface in us.

However, the two meanings of the term, usefully differentiated though they might be, are not fully separate, as each of us will resonate with each client a bit differently. Every therapeutic dyad is utterly unique. Our own backgrounds and emotional make-up equip us with a unique set of 'hooks' on which our clients can, and will, hang their own emotional and relational issues. Our completely individual personalities and histories – what Bollas (2018) and Coren (2009) refer to as 'idiom' – lead us to resonate with our clients in a highly specific way. Very disturbed clients might bring out similar dynamics in most people, although even then the impact will differ depending on who exactly we are.

As Mitchell (1993) puts it, 'The analyst is not a mirror, an inert object, but a complex meaning-generating subjectivity in her own right.' This subjectiv-ity is made up of both consciously remembered and unconsciously embedded elements, and will inevitably have its foundations in the particular personal development story of the individual practitioner. Thus the personal responses we have to our clients need to be understood in a range of ways: as coun-tertransference of the contemporary kind, i.e. an unconscious response to the relational dynamics brought into the work by the client; as the classical countertransference – i.e. the response to our client grounded in our own unre-solved conflicts and *our transference to them* and finally, as is explored at length in this book, as a response (both conscious and unconscious) to the way in which their presentation connects with our own experiences and sensibilities. While conceptually distinct, all three are likely to be involved to different degrees, and activated at different times, so the task of the counsellor – and supervisor – is to reflect on all three in order to make the most meaningful and useful sense of the dynamics that become evident.

Relational approaches

Alongside the changes in the ideas around countertransference, psychoanalytic and psychodynamic theory and practice have been changing in other ways, some of which have given rise to and been influenced by what is called the 'relational school'. These changes arise directly out of the acceptance that we are not a mirror, nor the fabled 'blank slate', and the acknowledgement that something much more complex is going on in the unique dyad. There are a number of issues here.

One relates to the relationship itself, and its role in helping our clients, while another relates to how much we do or do not tell clients about our own feelings and history. These might be seen to connect in many ways but they can and should be considered quite separately.

The role of the relationship

It has long been a central belief in psychoanalytic thinking that the relationship between therapist and patient IS the location of the work. It is through the relationship as it develops that the therapist gains the necessary depth of understanding of the client. For the client, it is through the experience of the relationship that they develop the capacity for a new relationship with themselves. In addition they build the ability both to perceive themselves and others differently and to behave differently with others. Change is facilitated not solely, not even primarily, through insight, even though insight is fundamental to the way the relationship works and is maintained. Rather, the way change comes about is through the experience of being with another person in this new and deeply significant way.

Mitchell (1993) highlights Benjamin's work on intersubjectivity (Benjamin 1992), pointing out her view that 'the full development of a sense of oneself as subject involves the search for recognition by another subject, that the full development of oneself as human entails a relationship to another whom one experiences as fully human.' Benjamin (ibid) stresses that 'Intrapsychic and intrapersonal processes are intertwined, and the enrichment of the analysand's subjectivity is arrived at through the establishment of a shared reality.' (p. 53)

In this approach to the work of therapy, the individuality of the therapist becomes much more vital and influential. If we resonate in a particular way with aspects of the material brought into the work by the client, our connections around these will intensify, creating a different kind of energy. In any child's growing up, certain aspects of their personalities will be noticed. In Benjamin's phraseology this is what it means to be 'recognised'; some traits encouraged and amplified by the family's reactions, some muted and stunted by being ignored or discouraged. Much of this will be unconscious, dictated by the unique emotional 'repertoire' of the family dynamics. This is not the same as the conscious policing of emotion in the family, nor the same as unconscious repression and driving of the unacceptable underground. It is more the ordinary way in which parts of us develop strongly and other parts never get brought out. I am mentioning it because a similar process happens in therapy. As Lemma puts it (2016): ' I have in mind here the inevitable disclosures of the real person of the therapist through the way we dress, talk, decorate our rooms, how much or how little we intervene, what we choose to focus on and what we may or may not laugh about with the patients.' (p. 121)

In any given therapeutic dyad certain aspects of the client will be more thoroughly brought into the light than others. Each therapist will emphasise different elements in their client, both at a conscious level through their formulations but even more powerfully at an unconscious level through their identifications and resultant preoccupations.

Therefore, as the chapters in this book will go on to explore more fully, our personal backgrounds and developmental stories, our unique blind spots and particular personal learning and insights, will play a crucial part in how we understand, respond to and engage with our clients. As Greenberg puts it, 'The suggestion that we can be blank screens or reflective mirrors seems a kind of conceit; the idea that we can judge and titrate abstinence appears arrogant and evenly hovering attention seems both epistemologically and psychologically naïve.' (1996 p. 212)

What we choose to explore

As indicated above, one element to pick out regarding the role of our own personalities and histories relates to what we choose to explore and what we ignore or at least fail to emphasise.

A New Yorker cartoon illustrates this in a characteristically quirky way. (Figure 1.1)

In the cartoon scenario, the psychoanalyst does not perceive that for the patient to have a cat on his head could be 'the problem' as he himself has a cat on his head. While we are not often confronted with clients with cats on their heads (!), we are all always at risk of not noticing something - or not thinking something is worthy of exploration and interpretation - if it resembles behaviour or opinions of our own. For example, if a therapist has a faith, she is less likely to be as closely attuned to or curious about what it means that her client believes in a similar way, while a therapist who is an atheist will think that there is a lot to try to understand in the meaning of the client's religious experience. If I have a client who is right-wing or pro-Brexit I will want to understand why and explore what drives them to have these views, while if he is broadly left-wing and pro-European, I might well just assume they are

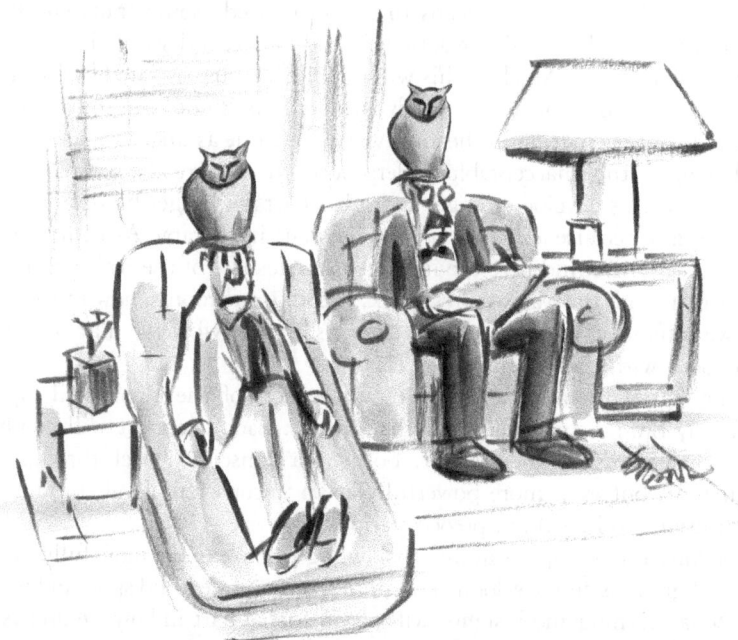

"So—what seems to be the problem?"

Figure 1.1 Lee Lorenz / The New Yorker Collection / The Cartoon Bank

sensible. If I care deeply about the environment I will think it worth analysing why my client is so resistant to taking steps to limit their carbon footprint, but if I am myself unmoved about these things I might want to analyse why my ecologically-minded client is so guilt-ridden. If I am vegan I might think my client thoughtful and 'right' to be so too, while if I am a meat-eater I might see it to be my task to analyse my vegetarian client's fear of their oral aggression.

In the 2020 pandemic we have had particular examples of this kind of problem, where our attitudes have been necessarily made explicit through the degree of caution with which we manage our practices. Clients who match our care will be seen as 'getting it' while those who want to break the rules or who seem to us overly cautious will be felt to need more understanding. These examples are fairly easy to spot and to get a grip on, but there are a multiplicity of subtler ways in which our own personalities and preferences will alter the tone and tenacity with which we address aspects of our clients' ways of thinking or being. With adolescents, we might respond differently to our promiscuous or gender-fluid client if we had a period of sexual experimentation and gender uncertainty in our own youth. If we took drugs and drank to excess in our teenage years we might be orientated in a different way to our clients' exploits in this area – whether this places us in a markedly anxious and admonishing direction or in one that is overly laid-back or even collusive.

So our own histories, idiosyncrasies and personal attitudes will be in play, even if we make conscious steps to stay as open-minded as possible. They will always influence the unique clinical dyad we create with our clients, and while we can work to mitigate any ill-effects this might have, we have to acknowledge it and accept that this is part of what we bring to the table.

Self-disclosure

A further area of controversy and contention in the counselling field is the issue of self-disclosure. If we *have* had similar experiences to those of our clients, or if we feel particularly strongly about something they are telling us because of our own backgrounds – we can accept that this affects the work but it is a further question whether we speak to them about it. Psychodynamic practitioners, compared with those from most other approaches, are particularly careful about this and tend to have much stricter rules about it. This is based on solid theoretical foundations which hold that the room for the client to freely to develop their idiosyncratic transference to us would be limited by factual information about us. For example, we make it difficult to be perceived as unable to be in a relationship if we let them know we are married with three children. And we prevent ourselves from getting access to the fantasies they have about us being privileged and utterly sorted if we readily share our struggles on becoming a functioning adult with some control over our lives. We need to know about our clients' versions of us – however unrealistic they may be - much more than they need to know about our real lives. Furthermore, there are risks with self-disclosure that we will burden them with our own problems or send out signals that we need them to go easy on us in certain areas. We might anger them with glib parallels we make between their situation and our own, or conversely they might assume that we understand their situation much better than we in fact do.

As mentioned earlier, they will know a lot about us from how we present ourselves – who we actually are with them. So there will always be aspects of our real selves evident, but the discussion on self-disclosure is more about whether we explicitly talk to them about our own experiences. There are adolescents with whom it can be very tempting indeed to let them know that we have been there and done that, just like them. They often assume, ancient as we may seem to them, that we had very staid adolescences. Many of us have been schooled by young people about how sexual relationships work these days, or how prevalent drugs are in their social lives, as if we could not possibly relate to the way they hook up with one another or indulge at a party. They can assume that we do not know what it is to feel excitement and desire with the intensity they do, or that we cannot possibly have been as lost or felt as broken as they do. They may not be able to imagine that we have ourselves failed exams, or have been excluded, or have hated our parents or made terrifying mistakes.

There may be cultural and societal assumptions made about us as well. I have had patients teach me eagerly what it feels to be an outsider, 'knowing' that I cannot possibly have felt this myself as I am so obviously part of the establishment. They will have no inkling that my own family experience of being Jewish and not feeling accepted in UK society runs deep in its makeup and emotional attitudes. While this may be a very pale version of what they are telling me about their own experience it can rankle that I am being seen as having always, effortlessly, 'belonged'.

In these circumstances we can find ourselves longing to tell them that we *do* understand from our own experiences. Adolescents may explicitly say that they don't feel comfortable talking to us about their experiences because they don't think we are going to be able to understand. That can tempt us into letting them know that we are not all that different, that we have survived what they are going through, that we got through it and so can they. At a more personal level we may bridle at the stuffy image they conjure up of us and want to assure them that we can relate to their feelings and are not that out of touch.

The mainstream psychodynamic attitude to this is to say that we need to work with this difficulty rather than wipe it away with a self-disclosure. If we start telling clients our stories we will have to work hard to discern what information about us means to them and indeed where to stop once we've opened that door. There is the risk of turning the spotlight onto ourselves rather than it being about them.

So while there may be occasions when to tell one of our own stories might be helpful, there will be many, many more when it is not. The chief question to ask ourselves, as always, is whether we are really saying things to promote the psychodynamic work or whether we are just making our clients feel temporarily better, or, even more importantly, making ourselves feel better. If we believe in working with the negative transference, we have to tough it out when clients feel unsure about or alienated from us. On the other hand there will also be times when the negative transference limits their ability to engage so much that they leave. Very careful judgement is needed and, as Lemma puts it 'In the vast majority of cases I can see no good rationale for (self-disclosure) from the vantage point of the best interests of the patient' (2016 p. 121).

Working with adolescents

The issues so far discussed are going to be in play whatever age-group we are working with. A therapist working with adults may have an added dimension of life experience which will pull on the connections with a patient's material. One patient of mine was struggling with parenting issues with her toddler in a way which felt very familiar to my own experiences, while another was bringing up their children in a way that I felt was so over-protective that I found myself becoming judgmental, maybe in defence of my own style of parenting. We might find our clients in marital tensions that painfully remind us of our own, leading us to closely identify with either them or their partners. However, this book encompasses work with adolescents and there is something uniquely powerful about this age-group which brings the issues discussed in the following chapters into a particularly sharp focus.

As mentioned earlier, we remember our adolescence in a way that we don't remember our childhood. It is a time when it is likely that we were ourselves in precarious positions and could easily have gone off the rails. While we are sitting in a room with our clients in the role of counsellor, we will know how close we came in times of crisis to sabotaging ourselves in a way that would have made our future professional roles as counsellors unrealisable. The risks we took, the traumas we faced, the bad decisions we made, the self-destructive defences we adopted (and often strenuously justified), the help we refused and the advice we ignored: all of these are still well within our own awareness and memory.

When we are working with adolescents there is always the anxiety-provoking knowledge that the stakes are very high. We are at a point where we might be able to play a part in influencing the young person's trajectory, either towards successful negotiation of their problems towards a rewarding adulthood or towards self-sabotaging manoeuvres which could seriously blight their futures or even end their lives. In these circumstances, the work evokes more vividly our own subjective experiences of navigating this period than when working with other age-groups.

The young people we work with often will be casting us in the role of 'another adult' at a time when adults have either actually failed them badly or are being perceived as doing so, and this might interfere with their capacity to use us well even if we are tuning into them more or less accurately. We are, much more than they might realise, likely to be identifying strongly with their struggles, still able to recall and, through them, relive, some of the dynamics that have shaped us in the past and can still reclaim us easily. This means that we need to work extra hard to sort out how to use our own subjectivity in the most effective way.

Phillips (2011) writes vividly about how much work with adolescents connects with our own experience: 'Working with adolescents gives us the opportunity to go on revisiting and possibly reworking the conflicts in our own adolescence; we may even hope to repair, vicariously, the things that went wrong for us'. 'The adolescents we see may … represent the disowned adolescent parts of ourselves. We may, that is to say, secretly recognise in these adolescents our own preoccupations about sex and solitude, and sociability; we may identify with them, and sometimes more than we want to.' (Ibid p. 190)

As Lemma puts it. 'In the course of any therapeutic relationship, we will experience temporary partial identification with our patients but our commitment is to relate to them as an 'other' and not be confused with ourselves. This requires vigilant monitoring of our own projections as the interaction that evolves between us and the patient is determined by unconscious forces operating in both'. (2016 p. 228)

We need to work hard on ourselves so that we can be optimally conscious of our own internal dynamics and be alert to how the client's material and presence is acting on us. We have to know our own stories as fully as possible, so that we do not get ambushed or misled by identifications which go undetected or take us by surprise. We need always to be sorting out where the energy of a feeling or a spur to action is coming from – is it theirs, ours or a complex mixture of the two? We need to pay serious attention to the 'real' relationship as well as to the transference, and to be acutely tuned into and honest about the way in which we co-create the shared reality of this unique dyad with our client. We can then be a bit more certain that we are making the best possible use of what we ourselves bring to the table, understanding how it helps us in making a good connection with the young person in front of us, but also vigilant to where it might be leading us astray.

As the chapters in this book will show, this is a difficult but rewarding set of tasks.

References

Benjamin, J. (1992). 'Recognition and destruction: An outline of intersubjectivity'. In N. J. Skolnick & S. C. Warshaw (Eds.), *Relational Perspectives in Psychoanalysis* (pp. 43–60). Analytic Press, Inc. (An earlier version of this chapter appeared in "Psychoanalytic Psychology," 1990, 7(suppl.): 33–47).

Bollas, C. (2019). *Forces of Destiny*. Abindgon: Routledge.

Carpy, D. (1989). 'Tolerating the countertransference: A mutative process'. *Integrated Journal Psychoanalysis*. 70 (Pt 2): 287–294.

Coren, A. (2001). *Short-Term Psychotherapy: A Psychodynamic Approach*. Basingstoke: Palgrave Macmillan.

Freud, S. (1912). 'Recommendations to physicians practising psycho-analysis'. *Standard Edition*. 12: 111–120.

Greenberg, J. (1996). 'Psychoanalytic words and psychoanalytic acts'. *Contemporary Psychoanalysis*. 32: 195–213.

Heimann, P. (1950). 'On counter-transference'. *International Journal of Psychoanalysis*. 31: 81–84.

Lemma, A. (2016). *Introduction to the Practice of Psychoanalytic Psychotherapy*. Chichester: John Wiley.

Mitchell, S. (1993). *Hope and Dread in Psychoanalysis*. New York: Basic Books.

Phillips, A. (2011). 'The pleasures of working with adolescents'. *Psychodynamic Practice*. 17(2): 187–197.

Racker, H. (1957). 'The meanings and uses of countertransference'. *Psychoanalytic Quarterly*. 26(3): 303–357.

Chapter 2

Stepping into the unknown

Reflections on transitions

Lyn French

Life is always lived in conversation with the past. Our perception of who we once were, who we are now, and who we are in the process of becoming draws on memories both remembered and 'forgotten', family histories told or unspoken, and the stories we create. Over time, these can be re-imagined or over-written, either knowingly or unconsciously, disguising or subtly distorting how things might have been. None of us can recall what has gone before with absolute precision; instead, we build internal pictures from a few memorable sequences, filling in the gaps with speculative imaginings and editing out as we go along what is seemingly too incidental, troubling, or painful to include.

As psychotherapists, we intuitively know that our memory is not simply a form of repository but a dynamic mental activity. Memory re-shapes recollections depending on the context in which we are recalling them as well as on any newly acquired knowledge. It can also be modified by, for instance, casting ourselves or our actions in a more favourable light or one more deserving of compassion. Neuroscientists support this idea, providing recent evidence showing that memories are reconstructed from scratch every time, using selected fragments of information which are then pieced together. Through research using brain-scanning, a network of regions has been identified as each having a part to play in determining what we remember, in what detail, and how vividly (Holmes, 2020; Yong, 2016).

Looking back with the benefit of many years of my own therapy, itself a process of gradually re-drawing the present in light of a more sharply defined past, late adolescence stands out as a particularly significant life phase. Although every generation has its challenges and a specific psycho-social landscape to navigate, the developmental tasks we all face in the transitional years leading to young adulthood remain more or less the same. The search for a new identity to replace the loss of our child self and the push towards independence evolves hand in hand with our growing awareness of having a mind within which we can think our own thoughts. If things have gone well enough, we develop a reflective capacity that enables us to become more conscious of who we are in relation to others. We start to question some of the beliefs we hold about ourselves and the world, introjected whole and undigested in infancy and

DOI: 10.4324/9781003270447-3

childhood. Acquiring an authentic sense of self depends on the ability "truly to suffer one's own experience in such a way that it may genuinely be learned from, rather than simply learned about or reacted to ..." (Waddell, 2018:26). Perhaps adolescence is such a tumultuous and confusing developmental stage because 'learning from' which sounds uncomplicatedly straightforward is often not. At least I have rarely found it so. Now with the distance that comes with age, I can pick out specific themes, some of which wind further back in time, weaving their way across different countries and earlier generations.

The yearning for a sense of belonging and the question of 'place in the world' are central strands in my story. I completed the equivalent of secondary school and Sixth Form in London before returning to Canada, my birth country, for university. I did this despite not being entirely certain where, or what, constituted 'home'. On the one hand, there was anticipatory excitement in striking out on my own, drawn as I was to the kind of independence that attending university further away entails. And on the other, being without a familiar base to reconnect with at weekends or term breaks was something untested and potentially daunting. I didn't allow myself to think too deeply about what lay ahead, nor was I encouraged to. Within my family, and at school, the transition to university, even to one in a different country, was treated as a natural step which everyone took; it didn't warrant attention other than sorting out the practicalities of where to apply and what to study. As I was a student at an American school in London, most of my peers were also leaving England. I imagine others, like me, might have felt ripples of fear and trepidation but such anxieties remained unspoken or perhaps for most, denied, as preparations for the graduation ceremony and parties to mark the occasion took over. In her book *Counselling Young People* (1983), Ellen Noonan, who had a seminal role in establishing student counselling services in universities in the UK, uses New Year's Eve celebrations as an everyday example of how, at times of transition, we try to circumvent the regrets and losses inherent in all endings, keeping our focus firmly fixed on the excitement of a new beginning. It is an apt metaphor for my perspective, or the absence of it, on the transitions I was to face.

I arrived in Canada just after my 18th birthday in a city chosen purely because it had been the last one our family had lived in before moving to London. This was just the first of what turned out to be a number of experiences of uprooting and transplanting myself elsewhere during my young adulthood in an attempt to find a place which felt a good enough fit. Although to the outside eye, and to a degree to my own, I was seeking new opportunities by transferring cities and universities more than once (something permitted in the Canadian system), I fleetingly sensed that my inability to fully settle had a more complex source despite lacking the knowledge or language to give this meaning or definition. From today's standpoint, I can see how my family's numerous moves due to my father's profession, first within Canada and then to London, were treated as functional, leaving in their wake much that remained unnamed and undigested. Vamik Volkan writes of how adolescence provides a model for an adult type of mourning as one must let go of childhood attachments. He goes on to say that immigration always involves gains and losses and that "dislocation from a familiar place to a foreign one leads to youngsters combining their internal and external turmoil, facing what Amsterdam-based psychoanalyst Jelly van Essen has called 'double mourning'" (Volkan, 2018:58). This can result in difficulty in adjusting to life and in consolidating identity formations. Experiencing a double mourning makes it hard to find a place 'in between' the culture and history left behind and those of the new country (ibid). Arriving in England, having never been before, was undoubtedly a more disorientating move for my family than had been anticipated. The fact that it was voluntary, and that the language was the same, left us unprepared for the task of adapting to a new culture with no support network to draw on and lacking the internal resources required to be able to talk about what we were going through both individually and as a family. One could say that returning to Canada as I did, alone in a now unfamiliar land, cracked open the crust of surface memory, allowing transgenerational experiences, never fully articulated or expressed, to push through.

As we now know, immigration trauma and trauma more generally can be passed down the line. Perhaps my attempts to find or create a sense of home were so perplexingly 'driven' and emotionally potent due to carrying traces of unprocessed trauma on both sides of my family. My own relocations can be seen to reflect those in my mother's life dating from the time she left home as a teenager until meeting my father in her late twenties just as hers, in turn, replicated aspects of her parents' dislocation. My maternal grandfather arrived in Canada aged six, travelling from Finland with only his mother, unusual for its time. To my knowledge, nothing is known of his father. At the tender age of three, my maternal grandmother experienced the death of her mother before leaving Finland for Canada when she was 17 to join her father. Who she lived with prior to reuniting with her father remains shrouded in mystery. Whether she made the long journey to Canada alone or with a companion has also been lost to history.

My maternal grandparents were part of Canada's third wave of immigration which peaked in the early 1920s with over 400,000 immigrants docking on ships from continental Europe. Canada began attracting Finns from the late 1880s onwards following the Russian Empire's 'Russification of Finland', an oppressive and wide-reaching policy aimed at ending Finland's political autonomy and subsuming Finnish culture and language. This first of two Russification campaigns triggered widespread Finnish resistance featuring petitions, strikes and passive resistance (which included resisting the draft) and eventually active resistance. As a result, vast areas of Canada became populated by Finns fleeing the harsher realities of life under Russian rule. Under the Canadian government's Dominion Lands Act, those who were willing to forego the urban centres were offered free land provided they agreed to build their own houses and cultivate their holding within three years (Wikipedia: various entries). It has been impossible to unearth the extent to which my ancestors' departure from Finland was motivated by personal as well as political or economic reasons, but the few facts known tell their own story. Whatever the context, the practical and emotional work involved in letting go of past attachments and establishing new ones would have been formidable.

Pioneering life in Canada was first captured in *Roughing it in the Bush* published by Susanna Moodie in 1852. I came across it when taking a course on Canadian literature as an option during my undergraduate degree. Moodie describes the sheer exhaustion resulting from clearing land and building houses as well as the kinds of tensions that could arise amongst the community of settlers. Her part-memoir, part-fictionalised account reveals a stark contrast between immigrants' expectations raised by the Dominion of Canada's advertising campaign and the day-to-day struggles they encountered. Regardless of country of origin, all of those arriving on Canada's shores in the first few waves of immigration left their homeland behind with many, like my grandparents, never able to return. One can imagine that these new homesteaders had little choice but to concentrate their efforts on survival which, for the most part, must have required blocking out their varied and many losses, turning away from the emotional hit of inevitable disappointments when reality collided with fantasy, and trying to dampen down the fear of being overwhelmed by the sheer enormity of the challenges they faced. In many instances, familial links were permanently severed once the ship set sail. Histories became half-forgotten or mythologised with the disowned parts, deeply buried, forming a layer of psychic sediment that could never lie entirely undisturbed in the generations to follow.

Back then, new arrivals tended to join their own communities with mutual dependencies rapidly evolving. This reliance on others – initially strangers – while not without complexities, allowed for a connection to one's homeland and the forging of strong bonds. Unlike the majority of first-generation Canadians who stayed within their kinship groups, my mother left hers as an older adolescent. Her life beyond the relative cocoon of what was then called 'New Finland' had distinct and often painful chapters, each taking her further from her childhood home, her mother tongue and her deep cultural links. By the 1950s, Canada prided itself on the emphasis it placed on integration which was predicated on overlooking or underplaying differences. Many preferred to believe that there was no clearly demarcated system of social class. However, like all societies, Canada featured social stratification from the start whether overt, such as in immigration agencies' advertising and related government policies, or oblique, as reflected in the way in which different nationalities were perceived as having higher or lower status. Immigrants from Britain and France secured the top ranking. My mother was keen to assimilate and identify as Canadian yet her history as a child of 'homesteader' parents from Finland, growing up in a closed community, speaking English as an additional language first learned in school and all that this symbolised never really left her, regardless of the distance she travelled internally and externally, educationally, and financially.

My father's family history ran on a different track. His paternal ancestors were linked to the Hudson's Bay Company (HBC) which still operates today. From its headquarters on the Bay, the HBC oversaw the fur trade for several centuries throughout much of what was then British-controlled North America. Those working as HBC managers, or 'factors' as they were called, functioned as the de facto government in many areas of Canada. My great-grandfather's diary recording his experiences in this role, including the complexities of establishing relationships with the indigenous First Nations tribes, now sits in a museum in Canada. My grandfather was the first in the family to leave the lucrative furrier business, relocating to Chicago to attend university, a move precipitated by the discovery that his birth father had died in an accident when he was an infant and the man who brought him up (his 'father') was in fact his uncle. Marrying a relative of a deceased husband was an acceptable although relatively uncommon practice. It kept the bereaved within the wider family network and provided economic security. However, learning this in his late teens, coupled with the new knowledge that he had been legally adopted by his uncle, came as a psychologically and emotionally loaded blow for my grandfather. The status of adoptee was one more commonly associated with illegitimacy making it an aspect of his identity that he fervently wished to disown.

Accommodating unexpected and difficult-to-assimilate knowledge of this kind usually involves dismantling the past and reassembling it piece by piece, a process that can be disturbing and destabilising. It seems the perceived betrayal and duplicitousness shattered my grandfather's world, leading him to turn his back on his family and move to the United States, only returning to Canada following completion of post-graduate studies and training in a medical field. I have no evidence, anecdotal or otherwise, of whether my grandfather's relationship with his mother and adoptive father/uncle was repaired, but the understanding is that it remained an open wound, affecting aspects of how he parented his own children. Tragically, my father's elder brother whose relationship with my grandfather was, from what little is known, complex and, no doubt, layered with projections, took his own life as a 17-year-old, an act that is difficult to separate fully from my grandfather's discovery of the death of his birth father at around the same age. This suicide remained a family secret about which I was told in confidence by a relative. I can still remember the shock I felt and the accompanying wish to 'unhear' it as soon as it had sunk in. It further complicated my no doubt still Oedipal-inflected picture of my father's family which, until that moment, I hadn't realised I had seen through my mother's eyes, unquestioningly placing them on an intimidatingly high pedestal due to my grandfather's medical background and my French grandmother's cultured ways. At the time, I was living on my own in Canada. When, on my next visit home, I shared with my older sister this piece of family history, by now corroborated by my father, it did not seem to hit her in the way that it had me, perhaps suggesting that I had a valency for 'receiving' the felt experience. This is just one example of how a story's emotional charge can reverberate through the generations, the telling of which conveys not simply the factual details but passes on at gut level that which has remained undigested. It shows, too, how we unconsciously take in the views of our parents, as, in this instance, I did my mother's.

My father's own late adolescence also featured leaving home in out-of-the-ordinary circumstances, derailing any opportunity of a more conventional progression out of school years into further studies. Coinciding with the early years of the Second World War, he joined the Canadian Air Force at 17, which entailed moving across the country first to train as a fighter pilot before heading abroad, returning to Canada at the end of the war and attending university on a fully funded government scheme for veterans.

A milestone in any adolescent's life is leaving home for the first time. This step on the developmental pathway is fundamental to the task of separating and becoming one's own person. My family history of late adolescent transitions is marked by emotionally freighted endings: my maternal grandmother departing Finland, ostensibly on her own; my paternal grandfather moving to the States for university, under the shadow of his recently discovered birth status; my mother leaving the safe haven of New Finland in the aftermath of the Great Depression to find work; and my father, signing up to fight in the war. All left in their wake unprocessed emotions and traces of trauma. The ruptures resulting from these kinds of endings are not healed by unconsciously repeating versions of them. Instead, disentangling and processing residual feelings and projections, which often involves detoxifying historical shame, allows us to arrive at a new understanding and to better accommodate and integrate what has gone before.

In common with many immigrants, I realised on my return to Canada that I felt neither fully at home there nor back in London. I chose to study fine art at university rather than at an art college so that I could also take more academic courses in art history, literature, and history of film. This was in part a semi-conscious response to what I intuited as my mother's complex feelings about her place in the world (and therefore mine as well) in relation to the higher status of my father's family line. My paternal grandmother spoke French fluently, was well read and interested in classical literature. Her set of Shakespeare plays ended up in pride of place on my bookshelf in my early teens when she died. The need to build 'cultural capital' was something I unknowingly absorbed by unconsciously tuning in to my mother's sense of lack, fuelling a wish in me to shore her up vicariously through my achievements. On the surface, my interest in art was as social as it was academic; at high school in London, I often spent time in the art room which was open at breaks, attracting those who were in some way different. That experience aroused curiosity about myself as well as about them. As it turned out, art took me somewhere I hadn't intended to go. On one level, looked at through the prism of my family history, making art may have been an unconscious attempt to fill the empty spaces left by the unknown stories of my maternal grandparents. There were neither photographs of them nor any type of 'artefact' which ordinarily serve as a material representation of a connection to those long gone, what Volkan named 'linking objects' (2018).

Another unconscious driver may have been the need to give form to or create an external container for what I can only describe as troubling 'felt experiences', perhaps linked to the unnamed multigenerational fear, anxiety, and other emotions connected to unresolved trauma transmitted down the line to me. The raw materials used in art making – canvas, clay, film, and so on – become both the medium with which the artist gives shape to ideas and the 'blank screen' onto which aspects of the psyche are unconsciously projected, whether in original or part-modified form. For me, although I could not fully understand it back then, this lent artmaking a particular type of anticipatory frisson. Beginning any new piece of art relies on a willingness to step into the unknown and tolerate unconscious material coming into the frame. It is never possible to predict what associations or thoughts might unexpectedly come to the surface or what kind of feelings previously disowned or disavowed might be triggered including the particular shame that threads through any kind of intergenerational trauma.

My uneasy relationship with artmaking was laced with uncomfortable-making questions: Do I have the right to 'be an artist'? Do I have something of value to say? Why is it so hard to accept what I make even when it is well received? The uneasy feelings and background chorus of questioning signalled something internal requiring resolution and a need to understand (although *what*, precisely, I didn't fully know). It contributed to my seeking therapy as a young person and eventually led to training, first in art therapy and then psychotherapy. The cumulative effects of therapy and training together provided the opportunity to defuse the power of the past. They have given me the capacity to identify and metabolise previously less tolerable emotional states requiring learning, unlearning, and re-learning, as well as developing the capacity to live with unanswered questions. I am reminded of Louise Bourgeois' inaugural exhibition (2000) at the Tate Modern in London. Entitled *I Do, I Undo, I Redo* it can be seen as a nod to a core task of therapy which facilitates using what Dan Siegel identified as 'mindsight': the capacity to monitor our feelings and thoughts, unpacking and disentangling them, and through this process modify our internal world. Neuroscience has shown that focusing our attention in these ways can actually change the physical structure of the brain (Holmes, 2020; Siegel, 2020).

Making art has been described by Bourgeois as her way of working and re-working themes from her childhood which preoccupied her in her own psychoanalysis and informed her thinking right up to the end of her long life. *I Do, I Undo, I Redo* comprised three imposing 30-foot-high rusted steel towers, two of which incorporated a narrow, tightly twisting staircase leading up to a platform jutting out at the top, seemingly suspended in air, surrounded by very large circular mirrors tilted at different angles. The third – *I Undo* – was a square tower also with an external spiral staircase and no platform to venture out onto but with a further staircase concealed inside. All three towers housed a bell jar containing sculpted figures of a mother and child. With those who wished to climb the towers limited to a few at a time, each person had to ascend on their own. Stepping out onto the 'floating' platforms of *I Do* and *I Redo* meant being on full and vulnerable-making view – via the giant magnifying mirrors – to those watching either from below or from the Tate's internal bridge spanning the Turbine Hall.

Bourgeois' powerful installation could be read as a metaphor for any significant transition when we experience a more acutely felt sense of self, heightened by being the object of our own gaze as well as that of others. Adolescence in particular brings with it the dawning awareness of having a mind within which we can step back and look at ourselves as well as witness being seen by others. Both states hold out the possibility of self/other acceptance or rejection, pain, or pleasure. For this reason, it is one of the most memorable phases of life for us all, more so if it coincides with other significant experiences such as moving city or country or if an event occurs that changes everything, such as a bereavement. Equally a shocking discovery can be destabilising and can threaten a derailment of adolescence, as my paternal grandfather discovered when he learnt that his 'father' was actually his uncle.

Binh, a 17-year-old client seen in a school-based counselling service, similarly faced difficult news which could have thrown her way off course. When she was referred to a therapist I was supervising, Binh was in her first term in the Sixth Form attached to her secondary school. An only child, she lived with her Vietnamese parents, both with their own complex histories of dislocation. They had made a life for themselves in their community. Binh's father worked as a chef in a Vietnamese café and her mother was employed full-time in a nail bar. Binh was a promising student with plans to go on to university, something her parents were very proud of. However, at the start of Year 12, Binh uncharacteristically began struggling to engage in her lessons, handing homework in late or failing to complete it. Her Head of Year thought Binh was showing signs of depression and suggested she try counselling. At first, Binh was reluctant to open up and was not able to say why her mood and motivation had both dipped so low. Careful exploration around her cultural background revealed that in her community, talking about personal subjects and private feelings with outsiders was actively discouraged. But once Binh had worked through what initially felt like a conflict of loyalties, she was able to relax and talk more freely.

Binh revealed that her mother had been diagnosed with bowel cancer and had gone through surgery the previous August with follow-on chemotherapy treatment set to continue until the end of January. The school had no knowledge of this. Binh said she'd been told the prognosis was good, but she had caught a glimpse of her mother sitting on the edge of her bed silently crying which unnerved Binh and caused her to question this. Binh couldn't bring herself to go in and comfort her mother, which left her feeling confused and riddled with guilt and shame. Instead, she went to her own room and texted an old boyfriend, Femi, with whom she had broken up over a year before. She had recently started a new relationship with Phong, also of Vietnamese heritage. Unbeknownst to Phong, Femi and Binh had continued to exchange short messages over the course of a term. Binh felt it was wrong to keep this up behind Phong's back and was only able to stop when Femi suggested meeting up, which panicked her. With the therapist's support, Binh was able to see herself more compassionately and understand that, at times of vulnerability, any of us can reach out, even if somewhat misguidedly, to old attachment figures. She was able to text Femi to let him know she'd met someone new and closed down the communication with him.

In Binh's second year of therapy some months after her mother had successfully completed her treatment and been signed off by the hospital consultant, Binh spontaneously remembered that Femi had once mentioned he'd been named after a much older stepbrother who had died of cancer in his twenties whom he'd never met. Binh's therapist helped her to see that even after the doctor had given her mother a reassuring 'all clear', she had been carrying an 'invisible loss' (Akhtar, 2020), that is, the unfounded but absolute conviction that her mother's cancer would return and she would die, based in part on what had happened to Femi's stepbrother. Contacting Femi the previous year, something that had been looked at with her therapist from many angles, now had a new context that reduced Binh's feelings of guilt and shame. Further exploration helped her to see that, as she was beginning preparations to complete Sixth Form and go off to another city for university, she really was about to lose her mother, that is, her 'childhood mother' upon whom we all depend from infancy into late adolescence. Over her time in counselling, Binh had gone through phases of feeling this impending separation and loss acutely. Gradually, she came to understand the emotional impact of leaving not only home but also letting go of some of her family's cultural beliefs and norms which felt to her a form of betrayal or disloyalty. However, she was able to face up to the fact that these were feelings and losses which had to be borne and, like her mother's cancer, were survivable, even if beginning the separation process was proving painful. She was able to achieve this state of acceptance through the benefits of longer-term therapy offered at just the right time and from having a secure network of caring others, including her parents who supported her decision to continue with counselling despite it being counter-intuitive to them. In addition, she had the backing of her Head of Year who recognised her emotional needs as well as her close friends and her boyfriend Phong and his family.

Late adolescence is characterised by the loosening of old ties and developmental, actual, threatened, or invisible losses which must be lived through. The independence we can both fervently wish for and fear in equal measure may be planned for and worked towards. Or it can feel like a blind leap of faith, sometimes driven by forces outside of our control; perhaps for all of us, it is a combination of both.

My focus has been on the internal upheavals of adolescent transition, carrying as it does the indelible imprint of the family's unique history and vulnerabilities. Although I have highlighted the inevitable losses and the impact of unprocessed transgenerational traumas, navigating such vicissitudes of adolescence sets in place the foundations for self-compassion, commonality, and empathy. We cannot protect our young clients from the pain of growing up, but we can offer them a space of open communication and close attentiveness that supports the development of 'mindsight' through which we co-create with them the kind of understanding which sparks a lively – even lifelong – curiosity about what makes us who we are.

References

Akhtar, S. (ed.) (2020) *Loss: Developmental, Cultural, and Clinical Realms*. London and New York: Routledge.

Artspace editors, '*I Don't Need an Interview to Clarify My Thoughts*': An interview with *Louise Bourgeois* by 22/08/2017 published online Artspace Magazine and Features www.artspace.com.

Cole, P. (2011) *The Uninvited Guest from the Unrememberd Past: An Exploration of the Unconscious Transmission of Trauma Across the Generations*. London: Karnac.

Cole, P. (2021) *Psychoanalytic Perspectives on Legitimacy, Adoption and Reproduction Technology: Strangers as Kin*. Abingdon and New York: Routledge.

Gismondi, M. (2020) The Untold Story of the Hudson's Bay Company commissioned by the Canadian Geographic commemorating 2020 in a series of articles, funded by the Government of Canada, celebrating milestone anniversaries of significance to the country's history. www.canadiangeographic.ca/article/untold-story-hudsons-bay-company.

Holmes, J. (2020) *The Brain has a Mind of Its Own*. London: Confer.

Siegel, D.J. (2020) *The Developing Mind: How Relationships and the Brain Interact to Shape Who We Are*. New York and London: Guildford Press.

Unilever Series: Louise Bourgeois: I Do, I Undo, I Redo https://www.tate.org.uk/.../unilever-series-louise-bourgeois-i-do-i-undo-i-redo.

Volkan, V.D. (2018) *Immigrants and Refugees*. Abingdon and New York: Routledge.

Waddell, M. (2018) *On Adolescence*. London and New York: Karnac.

Wikipedia: en.wikipedia.org/wiki/Finnish_Canadians; en.wikipedia.org/wiki/February_Manifesto; en.wikipedia.org/wiki/Dominion_Lands_Act.

Yong, E. *Memory Lane Has a Three Way Fork* pub.in Atlantic Magazine 25.10. 16 quoting research by Richter, F.R.*, Cooper, R.A.*, Bays, P., & Simons, J.S. (2016): Distinct neural mechanisms underlie the success, precision, and vividness of episodic memory. *eLife*, 5, e18260. (* joint first-authors).

Chapter 3

Shame, guilt, secrets, and lies

How differentness within and outside the family shapes our sense of self

Reva Klein

In my imagination the differentness of my family and of myself was a given, an understanding somehow internalised very early on in life. The nursery was crammed to the rafters with not only ghosts but with secrets, stifled sobs, and furtive whispers in strange languages (Fraiberg, 1975). As the first child of parents who, like so many, were desperate to repopulate a Jewish world that had been nearly obliterated in the Nazi genocide, I struggled to make sense of who I was supposed to be, what had happened 'over there' (Grossman, 1990), what it had to do with me and why I felt I didn't fit in to my family or indeed into the external world in which I found myself.

From the moment of my arrival, it felt as though I was assigned the role of my reincarnated paternal grandmother. This in itself isn't unusual or necessarily problematic in the realm of family scripts (Byng-Hall). But the brutal circumstances of her death, alongside the rest of my father's immediate family as well as the Jewish population of their Polish (now Ukrainian) village, conferred on her an idealised sacrosanctity and on me a projection of my father's magical thinking. Having been named after her and looking uncannily like her, there was the imperative that I would take on her legendary courage, goodness and intelligence. To this end my father executed his paternal function by trying to mould me into her image. The narrative around her superlative qualities could not be questioned. Instead, she was the ideal against which I was held up. Inevitably I failed time and time again. In a sense my father weaponised the 'perfection' of my murdered grandmother against my selfhood, my flawed self.

The result was a perfect storm: a clash between the development of my nascent ego and my father's desperate fantasies. I required, as all children do, unconditional love, a secure attachment and the space for individuation (Winnicott, Jung). As a flesh and blood human who made those demands known in the real world, my parents were ill-equipped to provide these conditions and became increasingly so.

There were significant reasons for this. My father's survival of the war was thanks to a Japanese diplomat who enabled him and two thousand other Jews to get safe passage to the Shanghai Ghetto, a refugee camp run by the

DOI: 10.4324/9781003270447-4

International Red Cross which at the time was under Japanese occupation. The privations and disease endured in this camp were considerable, as were his survival instincts. He had cousins who had left Poland in the 1920s and settled in the US, from where they'd been continually frustrated in their attempts to bring him over. Due to anti-Jewish immigration policies in the US after the war, it was seven years before they managed to bribe a congressman to arrange an American visa for him in 1949. He finally arrived in the US full of hope but ravaged by guilt and grief at having left his family and his village to their fate.

For her part my mother was born in America to Ukrainian Jewish immigrants. Yiddish was her mother tongue. She experienced the loss of her father and poverty during the Depression and was forced to leave school in her early teens to help support the family. For the rest of her life she, like my father, was haunted by anxious memories of hunger and both of them developed disordered eating, resulting in obesity. She was bedevilled, too, by low self-esteem due to, among other things, her lack of education. Eventually she resolved to study hard and achieved her high school equivalency diploma in her mid-50s, once her children had left home.

How they internalised their life experiences before marriage left them overwhelmed as parents of four children. Compounding these problems was the fact that each of the three daughters who arrived after me at two yearly intervals presented with impairments or conditions – neurological, cognitive, and/or physical – that made them fragile and in need of special attention. The sister closest to me in age had rheumatic fever in infancy and was considered 'delicate', the one after her was labelled 'mentally retarded' due to oxygen deprivation at birth as well as having undiagnosed Asperger's. The youngest was in and out of hospital for numerous surgeries after contracting polio.

As the only one of four spared my sisters' challenges, my health came at the cost of not appearing to need the attention that the others did. I acquired a second skin rather quickly and I needed it (Bick, 2018). The effects of my father's wartime traumas and survivor guilt manifested in violence against me: emotional, physical, and verbal. And my mother's withdrawal into depression in the face of her children's myriad difficulties, added to her husband's volatility, led her to become what I would understand many years later a 'dead mother' (Green, 1999).

My otherness within the family and the unrelenting Sturm und Drang in the household combined to create a theory of mind in which I also felt different from people outside my family throughout my childhood and adolescence. The microculture of my home was wildly at odds with the mom-and-pop imagery of white mid-century America where the sun always shone and families were happy, where jokey fathers without strange accents played baseball and mothers were glamourous and easy-going. It clashed with the discord, rage, unarticulated grief and foreignness that I was entrenched in. The tragic family history that could not be spoken about as well as the very present mental ill health of my parents and their children's various difficulties put us firmly outside the norm that I saw around me, or that I imagined existed.

To my shame now I felt ashamed of the collective strangeness of my family in contrast to my friends and cousins who had families that appeared to be calm and happy, in which people spoke respectfully to each other. I was also embarrassed at being in the only observant Jewish family at my schools throughout my education. This meant packed kosher lunches and missing school to go to synagogue for holidays that nobody else, including my non-observant Jewish friends, had ever heard of. When I was in the second grade I had my bottom paddled by my teacher for my frequent absences. My mother's protest at Mrs Hall's anti-semitism only amplified my sense of being out of synch with the rest of the world. It's only with hindsight that I have come to respect and been proud of my mother for challenging the school.

These combined factors led me, from the age of around nine onwards, to spend more and more time staying with friends and cousins who understood my need to escape. Only after a decade of therapy many years later was I able to see ironic echoes of my acts of self-preservation with those of my father.

One of my strongest positive memories of life with my family was a different kind of reality, a version of Lacan's pain-in-pleasure concept of jouissance (2007). It was the exhilaration of terror generated by the frequent tornadoes we would get in springtime. The sky would darken to deep purple as the hot, heavy air became unnervingly still. And then the screaming wind and battering of the windows would come for what seemed like hours. The haunting wail of the alert to take shelter and the all-clear afterwards was sounded by an air raid siren, nerve-jangling and thrilling at the same time. Part of the intense excitement and pleasure I experienced, I now understand, came from knowing that these extraordinary, oddly sensual phenomena were totally external and impersonal, experienced by *everybody*: an oddly comforting relief from the targeted tempests within the family. Similar to the threat of nuclear war – a very real fear in my early childhood – it was a shared experience, something that I couldn't be blamed for; not dissimilar to the oddly comforting oneness I felt with millions of unknown others during lockdown.

I also couldn't be blamed for being white and therefore privileged in what was then and remains one of the most racially segregated cities in the United States. But guilt was there nevertheless. It was just a little over 100 years since my home state of Missouri, half Confederate and half Union, had been forced to emancipate slaves, but black people were still openly referred to in derogatory terms at home, in my extended family and by many classmates. Growing up at the height of the civil rights movement, the only black children I ever saw were a handful of fellow students, the vast majority of whom were internally segregated, allocated to a separate class together with children with special needs. They lived in the suburban black ghetto about two miles and a world away from my white neighbourhood. Back then there were few paved roads in their streets of what were called crackerbox (tiny cramped) houses. Social mixing was unheard of with these children and the only time we inhabited the same general space was in PE and lunchtimes. I was curious about the black kids and their lives outside of school. At some level that was never acted upon I felt drawn to them *because* they were different. The attraction to people on the outside would lead me into my first (and top secret) relationship with a boy who was of Native American heritage at the age of 15.

But as opposed to people of colour, my differentness was invisible, something I carried inside me. There was nothing that externally marked me out as being, in the eyes of the world, less-than or threatening in the way African Americans' blackness brought them. My whiteness conferred on me membership into the mainstream to which I felt I didn't belong. Fortunately I had very close friends who, for different reasons, also saw themselves as different. On our roller coaster ride through adolescence we rebels with various causes grew increasingly creative, curious, and risk-taking.

Coming from these experiences, the questions of identity and of how we perceive ourselves and believe others perceive us led me, many years later, to immerse myself in psychotherapy trainings and personal therapy. Being exposed to psychoanalytic theory and research and thinking about attachment theory as well as intergenerational guilt and trauma came as much a relief to me as those tornadoes did in their different ways (Mucci 2013, Karpf 1996). I realised I was not alone. There were reasons, shared by many others, for my sense of alienation, self-denigration, and the desperation to become separate.

There was further clarity when eventually I learned about my father's experiences and those of his family. The information came mainly from other relatives and old friends of his from the resistance movement in which he was heavily involved in Poland. It helped to make some sense of the ghosts, the secrets, the cries in the night, the violence, and the depressive withdrawals, all of which had left their long shadows and indelible marks on my consciousness and my unconscious.

In working through my own internalised experience as the insider/outsider, one of many things that has become clear is that intense screen memories, shot through with fantasy, are the unreliable witnesses to the past and at the same time one of the foundation stones for the narratives we tell ourselves about where we have come from literally and emotionally. The extent to which we have choices about what we do with these memories or more precisely, these impressions, and ultimately about the way we define ourselves is inestimable. So too is the potential of psychotherapy to co-create a space in which these crucial challenges and adjustments to our clients' sense of self can develop.

An appreciation of this has become increasingly present in my relationally oriented clinical and supervisory work and the centrality of the concept of intersubjectivity to this way of working. The intersection of minds

> allows [us] relentlessly to seek a dialogic form of empathic understanding with the patient, to acknowledge and explore our mutual participation in the psychological field we develop together and thus to create a "developmental second chance" for people whose early and later lives have crushed and terrified them into aggressive and/or passive means of self-protection.
>
> (Orange, 2009)

Donna Orange promotes the placing of intersubjectivity into a 'systems theory' frame, giving it form and a place among other theories. It is a concept that reflects what this book essentially sets out to explore:

> the view that personal experience always emerges, maintains itself and transforms in relational contexts.... As a clinical sensibility it primarily includes an emphasis on the emotional convictions or organising principles that systematise experience, the personal engagement of the analyst and the refusal to argue about reality.
>
> (Orange, ibid)

Like so much in psychoanalytic thinking, intersubjectivity has lent itself to subtly varying but complementary definitions. Daniel Stern describes the intersubjective self as 'a stage and process of recognition of another's subjectivity as connected and responsive to one's own' (1985). Elaborating on this idea further, Jessica Benjamin stresses the centrality of mutual recognition to the development of intersubjectivity, where 'the subject gradually becomes able to recognise the other person's subjectivity, developing the capacity for attunement and tolerance of difference' (Benjamin, 1990).

To me a particularly useful aspect of intersubjectivity is the way it offers us, among other things, a way to think about the heavy psychic baggage of our backstories that we carry into and sit with in the consulting room. And indeed everywhere. It puts paid to the inhibiting notion of the blank slate. In its stead it allows us our humanity with all its complexities in a relationship with another complex human, together and separately, always with the understanding that we are products of and inextricably linked to the systems we have come from and in which we operate.

In a school context this begs the question of how the mental space we think of as thirdness finds room to allow for two peoples' individuality and agency when we work as a system within a system, contained within an intricate organisation with its own tight structures. Within this frame, we are not only adjacent to the school culture, to which we invariably have our own historical transferences based on childhood or experiences as parents, but we are also met with staffs' interpretations about the children and young people we see. Client referrals coming from teachers or inclusion managers communicating their own subjectivities overtly or subtly is often where we start thinking about the young person. And then there are our own responses to the referral details, however minimal they may be. This means that before we ever lay eyes on the new client there are already associations and transferences, conscious and un-conscious, to the referral itself and to how it is constructed. Then there is our own processing of information or inferences on clients' gender/gender identity, ethnic/cultural/socio-economic background, family circumstances, age, and even their name.

Inevitably there are challenging, stimulating, and illuminating clinical sce-narios that can arise when the client's narrative has resonances to our own. These situations carry the potential of powerfully drawing us in by strong countertransference and even projective identification. It can also usefully pro-vide a fertile ground for recognition, for 'being able to connect to the other's mind while accepting [their] separateness and difference' (Benjamin, 2007).

This was the case with one of my early clients, a boy I'll call Azad, who I worked with on and off from Year 9 to Year 11. His parents, before their four children were born, had come to the UK as refugees from Iraq. The referral for counselling was driven by teachers' concerns that he was disengaged and underachieving and that he presented with low mood due to a sibling's life-threatening illness. One teacher was concerned that his state of mind made him a likely candidate for 'radicalisation'.

Despite his poor hygiene, ungainliness, and initial monosyllabic mutterings, or perhaps *because* of these things, I felt there was something compelling about Azad when we had our initial meeting. The framing of his story as an outsider within his family and in the wider world pulled me in with stronger echoes to my own story than I had been aware of at the time.

While first distrusting me for being part of what he saw as the persecutory institution of the school and the white privileged world it represented, he grad-ually warmed to the idea of having someone he could offload onto. And offload he did, unwrapping little by little the story of his family but also the story of the culture he was born into and was both drawn to and resentful of. Entwined in his narrative was the story of a country that shaped his identity but was 'primitive' and 'filthy' in contrast to London, where he'd been born and raised.

Azad's parents had fled their country with nothing but the proverbial clothes on their backs. His father had had some involvement in the resistance move-ment against the regime. They left behind, as refugees usually do, everything they had and had known: their parents and extended family, their culture and property, and the father's good job, heading for a future that was full of un-knowns. Once settled in London the father managed to buy a small corner shop where he worked long hours. The couple had four children, two boys and two girls.

Fast forward 15 years to Azad's first year at secondary school when his oldest brother became seriously ill. The parents froze. The traumas of fleeing their home and their continued struggles to acculturate to life in the UK were now compounded by the existential threat to their first born. Their focus became concentrated on their son's survival and Azad, as the next oldest among the four children, was handed the responsibility to interpret at medical appointments and to help with his brother's care after school and at weekends. While filled with anxiety and compassion for his ambitious, high-achieving and now desperately ill brother, Azad guiltily acknowledged his resentment of him and even more so, of the parents who now appeared disinterested in his own struggles. While he had excelled in primary school, the transition to secondary school and the circumstances of his brother's illness dragged him down. His parents' sense of beleaguerment and defeatedness took root in him, leaving him struggling to adapt to his strict new school full of new people, new procedures, and new challenges. There was, he felt, no comfort in his world.

The work with him deepened as his disaffection with life grew. He expressed his need for an identity and his yearnings took the form of romanticising the same Iraq that he also denigrated. His desire was stirred for something different, dramatic, and outside his lived experience, an association with a place or an idea that would afford him a way of defining himself positively, an identity that his parents had had stripped away from them when they were forced to leave their country.

Throughout our sessions we explored his conflicted sense of self as 'a Hackney boy' who spoke Arabic and ate Iraqi food but who felt invisible except as an extra pair of hands at home. He felt as out of place in the mosque as he felt in the school playground. With time I came to feel a strong association with him drawn on my own experiences of growing up in a household that was riven with struggle due to historical and present circumstances, of feeling alienated from the religious observances I was coerced into following and with my own needs sidelined in favour of my sisters' more pressing ones.

My role, my thinking, and my feeling around the work with Azad gained further intensity when his mother asked to see me. Throughout most of the three or four consultations with her over a period of a school year she wept and, in her minimal English, expressed her fears, anxieties, and guilt about her sick son, about Azad's unhappiness, and about leaving her birth family behind. I felt drawn in to her projections of helplessness and grief. There was an uncomfortable familiarity about her distress and my intersubjectivity tipped over into over-identification with her. I was only able to fully understand the extent of this in supervision, where I had the space to confront my urge to rescue Azad and his mother. Through working with my supervisor and in my own therapy I was able to reposition myself and adapted Bion's 'no memory, no desire' to fit this particular situation. I had to reposition my own backstory and emotional needs back in their place, outside the frame, to stop it from interfering with the work. Rather than submitting to an impulse to rescue these people,

I concentrated on listening and communicating my interest, curiosity, and understanding, thereby offering some containment. I also suggested to the mother how she might get emotional support for herself via her GP. With time, the intensity of Azad and his mother's hunger for recognition and/or deliverance moved into a more circumspect mental space on both their parts. And I too could be more circumspect about my role and the boundaries that are so crucial to our work.

Azad continued the therapy on and off until he started his A levels. His low mood and confusion about himself were sublimated into working hard and in the summer he dropped me a line to let me know he was considering an offer from a top London university.

That early experience was a salutary and influential one in terms of illuminating the compelling nature of unconscious pulls into the role of rescuer. Narcissism and altruism are very companionable bedfellows which can come together synchronistically. The work with Azad sensitised me to my valency for wanting to repair clients' damaged psyches in an unconscious bid to rewrite my own family history.

More recently I've been working for several years with an Albanian woman, Yeta, who brought another deeply resonant issue to the therapy. She had come in a state of desperation due to her inability to form a meaningful and sustainable romantic relationship with a man. She had had a few months of CBT following the end of an abusive relationship a year earlier which she saw as a gateway therapy to something more in-depth. She was in her late 30s and was feeling the pressure to find someone lovable and loving who wanted to have children with her. I was moved by her longing but it was the unfolding narrative of being the focus of attention of her tyrannical father that opened up an intersubjectivity between us that I hadn't anticipated.

Yeta was, to the outside world, an enviable human being. A microbiologist who had risen to a high professional standing following a stellar academic career, she also had dazzlingly glamorous good looks. But she was lonely – despite her very wide circle of well-heeled friends – and felt there was something about her that made women dislike her and that also either pushed men away due to her Ice Queenly defences or ignited in them a desire to possess and dominate her. She came to therapy on the recommendation of an English friend who suggested there was some unearthing of her early life experience to be done before anything could change. How right that friend was.

There was considerable resistance at first, something that felt at times like an existential struggle within her fighting against loosening her defences and allowing her vulnerability to come through. For her, vulnerability was a moral deficit. As a scientist, she held on to the familiar world of objectivity and rationality, wanting answers to questions about what therapy could do and how it worked, questioning what we were doing, what could possibly change for her. To the many questions I would reflect back on her desire for certainties and her fear of being seen. I told her we were working towards co-creating a different kind of space where she could *be* and be heard and where she could see more clearly the patterns of behaviour and thought that were problematic to her. I said this despite being buffeted by doubt myself that it would ever happen. It took long months and the death of a beloved grandmother before she was able to engage on a more emotionally authentic level with the work.

Yeta's narrative unfolded as an Oedipal struggle that was framed within the context of the totalitarian regime in which she grew up for the first 11 years of her life and which continued to cast a shadow long after it was toppled. Her father was a latter-day Thomas Cromwell, Henry VIII's right-hand man as imagined by Hilary Mantel: brutalised as a boy by his father and the harsh politics of the time, mired in terrible poverty and determined to one day be rich and powerful through sheer ruthlessness. Her father achieved his wish but at the cost of alienating his birth family, his wife, and his two daughters. Yeta, the oldest, was her father's narcissistic trophy: clever, beautiful, wanting nothing more than to shine, doing everything she could to win her father's approval. But her father reproved rather than approved, determined to mould her into his paradox-ridden idea of perfection: she had to be scholarly and sporty, asexual and womanly, intellectually active, and emotionally submissive. She grew up confused and bruised by his constant criticisms of her. Instead of praising her for her 99% on exams he would angrily demand to know what happened to the 1% she had 'failed' at. When she wore clothes that accentuated her beauty, he would insist she put on something that neutralised her. When she started enjoying and excelling at swimming he made her give it up to concentrate on her cello lessons, which she loathed. Never was there a celebration of her achievements or a concession to her desires. His need to control her was matched only by her yearning for his love and approval.

Alongside her father's hypervigilance to her throughout her childhood and adolescence, Yeta witnessed her mother being denigrated and emotionally abused by her husband. The young girl introjected the idea that her mother, who had practised as a GP before having children, was worthless, weak, and unattractive, a quintessentially negative role model for her. Yeta had internalised the view that potency and strength were to be aspired to and that vulnerability was something to be despised. Her low estimation of her mother was amplified when her mother made several suicide attempts as a result of her husband's various affairs. The mother's severe depression led to her going to her parents in another town to be looked after, taking the younger daughter with her. During that two-year period of the mother's absence Yeta was sent away to stay with other relatives, about which she has little memory apart from seeing her father only intermittently and pining for him.

When the family came together again there were often angry scenes between the parents followed by silent withdrawals. Yeta survived by burying herself in her studies and her various lessons and sports outside of school. After finishing secondary school she left home to study abroad, totting up three degrees at prestigious universities across Europe. As for her father, as he grew older his desire to retain control over her waned but was reactivated, reaching new heights when he insisted she stay in a marriage to a French man. Having a western son-in-law may have been a huge status symbol to him, but the French husband was a source of deep unhappiness to Yeta. Her will prevailed and the divorce went through, resulting in a rupture between daughter and father that remains to this day. It also led Yeta soon after into a two-year abusive relationship with a man who wanted to possess and dominate her. It ended with her feeling utterly broken, in her words, and homeless in every sense.

These revelations emerged little by little as we worked through the buried material in her unconscious. It was jarring for her to come to realise the extent of the influence her father had on her, how hungry she had been for his love and how, unconsciously, she repeated aspects of that fraught entangled web with him both in her friendships with women and in romantic relationships with men. In all her relationships, including with me initially, she felt guarded, sensing people were poised to betray or manipulate her. So she kept women at arm's length and with men, she would get pulled in to their desire to own her and at the same time felt terrified of becoming submerged in their fantasies of who she should be. So she would retreat, alone again.

It was similarly jarring for me to see how the ferocity of her father's love for her had been perversely twisted into a controlling narcissism in which his own needs superseded hers. It was familiar, too familiar, and at times I had to metaphorically hold onto my seat, struggling to evoke the third position as she expressed the different ways the relationship with her father had affected her. I was furious with this bully who had himself been mercilessly bullied by his own father. And the rage against my own bullying father, something that I thought I'd worked through in my therapy was now being reignited since his death. I was unprepared for the strength of my feeling because, following my father's descent into dementia, I had finally been able to feel and show the compassion and sadness for him that had eluded me for so long.

Yeta is certain there will never be resolution in her relationship with her father and that this will continue to influence her lack of success with men. Her father has taken to raging against the dying of the light (Thomas, 1951) that comes with the territory of ageing despots among others, and her occasional visits to her parents ultimately lead to eruptions with her father when they can no longer stick to anodyne pleasantries or avoidance of each other. Her relationship with her mother, too, remains one of deep discomfort for her because of the collusion with her husband that her mother has chosen to follow in order to keep the peace and the status quo. What her mother has gained in social and financial security continues to come at the expense of her mental health, not to mention her relationship with her firstborn.

Yeta chose to end the therapy after the 2021 summer break. She was feeling battered and bruised after a few weeks with her parents, feeling that nothing would ever change, least of all herself. She insisted it was a pause, that she wanted to see what it was like to be without our weekly sessions after four years.

I affirmed and supported this pause, telling her that there are always arguments for ending just as there are for continuing. But I felt that at this point, her defensive portcullis had firmly shut and that she couldn't or wouldn't raise it for the time being: the light that beckons on the other side feels too harsh, the air too raw. The siren call of her psychic retreat has beckoned too irresistibly.

It goes without saying that I have asked myself whether Yeta perceives of the therapeutic relationship with me as yet another failure in a long line of them. But based on what she said in the run-up to our ending she was clear that she experienced the therapy as a singular relationship in her life. It has been, she said, one that has helped to contain some of her anxieties about herself, her present, and her future and that has enabled her to make connections between her insecure attachments in childhood and her difficult relationships in adulthood. She has come to accept that relationships are dynamic and that the unconscious leads us into transferences, into projections, and into reacting to the projections of others in ways that can't necessarily be acted on in the moment but can be understood and modified through that understanding. She has experienced this relationship, she said, as a very different kind of coming together. I would concur with that, having confronted my own emotional triggers, not for the first time, in my clinical work.

In writing about my work with these two clients I have been struck again and again by something that we all know from before we even begin our trainings but that we can sometimes forget in the busy day-to-day clinical pressures we work under. And that is how, as therapists, our foundations in the work are informed as much by our own subjective experiences of life as they are by the theories we draw on to give our thinking structure, depth and dimensionality. That we learn from each therapeutic relationship is irrefutable. Each is unique and adds more prisms into the kaleidoscope of our perceptions. That we learn about *ourselves*, our persistent fault lines despite sometimes many years of therapy, is something that, if we're open to those revelations, is invaluable to us as human beings as well as practitioners. Understanding those fault lines through reflection on our own and in supervision can lead to further opening up of our thinking, both in our personal worlds and in our clinical work.

References

Benjamin, J. (2007) *Intersubjectivity, Thirdness and Mutual Recognition*. Lecture at The Institute for Contemporary Psychoanalysis, Los Angeles, CA.

Bick, E., Harris, M. (2018) *The Tavistock Model: Papers on Child Development and Psychoanalytic Training*. Harris Meltzer Trust, London.

Bollas, C. (1999) Dead Mother, Dead Child, in Kohon, G. (ed) *The Dead Mother: The Work of Andre Green*. 87–109. Routledge in association with the Institute of Psychoanalysis, London.

Byng-Hall, J. (1985) The Family Script: A Useful Bridge between Theory and Practice. *Journal of Family Therapy* Vol. 7 301–305.

Fraiberg, S., Adelson, E., Shapiro, V. (1975) Ghosts in the Nursery: A Psychoanalytic Approach to the Problems of Impaired Infant-Mother Relationships. *Journal of the American Academy of Child Psychiatry* Vol. XIV 387–421.

Green, A. (1999) *The Dead Mother: The Work of Andre Green.* New Library of Psychoanalysis, London.

Grossman, D. (1990) *See Under – Love.* Washington Square Press, New York.

Karpf, A. (1996) *The War After: Living with the Holocaust.* New Hampshire: Heinemann.

Lacan, J. (2007) *The Ethics of Psychoanalysis Book VII: The Seminar of Jacques Lacan.* 194. Routledge Classics, London.

Mucci, C. (2013) *Beyond Individual and Collective Trauma.* 41–48. Karnac, London.

Nayar-Akhtar, M.C. (2019) 'There Is No Baby without a Mother' – Donald Winnicott. *Institutionalised Children Explorations and Beyond* Vol. 6, No. 2 113–117.

Orange, D. (2009) Intersubjective Systems Theory: A Fallibilist's Journey. *Annals of the New York Academy of Sciences* Vol. 1159, No. 1 237–248. New York.

Thomas, D. (1951) *Do Not Go Gentle into that Good Night.* Botteghe Oscure, Rome.

Urban, E. (2005) Fordham, Jung and the Self: A Re-examination of Fordham's Contribution to Jung's Conceptualisation of the Self. *Journal of Analytical Psychology* Vol. 50, No. 5 571–594.

Chapter 4

Feeling dislocated

Some personal and clinical reflections on the experiences of relocated families

Angie Doran

Introduction

I was the youngest of four children, all born in the Malay Peninsula. My parents had moved from London, starting their married life there in the early 1950s nearly a decade before I was born. By uncovering my own memories in personal therapy, I have become more conscious of the relationships, associated feelings, and experiences of my childhood. And by reflecting on my parents' personal histories, aided by reading letters written by my mother to my maternal grandparents, I have come to better understand aspects of my mother's emotional experience of raising four children in a foreign country. It's important to say that the perspective I hold of my childhood is my own; my three siblings will have their own memories and each may have different felt experiences of our shared family life.

In this chapter I reflect on my parents' story of relocation to a very different environment and the impact this had on their approach to parenting and the family they created. I do this with reference to my own story and with the stories in mind of many of the young people I've worked with. I focus mainly on my mother's experience of moving to a new country as, for reasons that will become clearer, these are most available to me.

My parents' migration story

Both my parents were of Irish heritage, born to first-generation immigrants living in London in the 1920s. My mother's father was a travelling salesman and my father's, a Post Office employee; my grandmothers both worked at home, as housewives. My mother left school with a good head for numbers and started work at the Bank of England. My father joined the British army after leaving school. In February 1942, my father was captured in Singapore following a ferocious battle between the British and Japanese armies, and he subsequently spent more than three years in a prisoner of war camp subjected to forced labour, building the Burma 'Death Railway' as a military captive. My father was just about 25 years old when World War Two ended and he was released and repatriated to

DOI: 10.4324/9781003270447-5

England in Autumn 1945, three months after VE Day. After a while, back in the UK, he found employment as a clerk in a north London bank. My aunt, his sister, worked alongside my mother at the Bank of England. She introduced my parents and over time they became engaged.

In 1948, a regular bank customer offered my father a job as the assistant manager of a rubber plantation in pre-independence Malaysia. My father jumped at the chance to return to Southeast Asia, the same region of the world where he had been wounded as a soldier and subsequently endured several years of torture, starvation, brutality, and disease as a prisoner of war.

The concept of repetition compulsion may help shed some light on my father's pull back to Asia. As therapists we may work with clients who describe 'the compulsion to repeat' (Freud 1920/1961), a process by which some people find themselves psychologically drawn to revisit the scene of their trauma. According to Freud, the patient "is obliged to repeat the repressed material as a contemporary experience instead of .... remembering it as something belonging to the past" (Ibid.:12). One understanding of this is that by returning psychically to the scene of their distress, the survivor is unconsciously creating for him or herself opportunities to overcome or 'master' those traumatic experiences by achieving a different outcome.

In the late 1940s, Britain was still clinging to the final phase of its role as a dominant world power at the same time as being driven to rebuild itself after the War. On the other side of the globe the Federation of Malaya was one of the world's biggest producers of tin and rubber, materials crucial to the reconstruction challenges Britain faced at the time. Encouraging young people to emigrate to its far-flung territories was an important part of Britain's post-war programme. There was a widely held view that Britons could relocate, settle, and become integrated anywhere within the Empire; that they would find 'their people' and that the colonies were theirs to command. There was little anticipation of trouble around assimilation or developing a sense of belonging. For my young parents, the idea of moving six and a half thousand miles across the world was no doubt anxiety-provoking, but above all it was an adventure. The belief was that there would be no need to adjust or change their cultural assumptions in any significant way. And so they moved, my mother following my father after a period of about two years, into a ready-made community, representing a particular kind of British life transported to the Far East.

Strong parallels and sharp contrasts: my story and my clients'

Like other psychotherapists based in London state and academy schools, I see a significant number of young people from migrant backgrounds. In our work together, we explore their parents' experiences of their newly adopted country, as well as the emotional tensions that exist with regard to the country of origin, including the important relationships that have been left behind. Their parents' experiences are the emotional foundations of my clients' early years and these stories shape their young psyches. Many of my clients are children whose parents have been the first of their family to settle in this country for economic reasons or to find political asylum. Like my parents, these people from countries such as Poland, India, Pakistan, Afghanistan, Nigeria, Bangladesh, Vietnam, Romania, and Yemen have moved across the world with a combination of high hopes and trepidation. The stories of family movement that I hear in the consulting room are of migrants relocating into a patchwork of relationships with people from their home country. Perhaps an uncle, a sibling, or a cousin had settled here and was able to offer somewhere to live initially or, as was often the case, they arrived knowing no one. Their tales are of extreme financial hardship, fractured family relationships, exclusion through language, and tremendous hard work.

For the majority of my young clients' parents it has taken some time to establish themselves in the UK. In contrast, my parents arrived into a fully formed colonial community, with all the sense of entitlement that this offered. My parents' new life featured fancy dress parties, anniversary balls, dinners at the club, golf and tennis, swimming pools, and servants: the standard trappings and social codes of a wealthy lifestyle embraced by white expatriate communities abroad after World War Two. My family had a gardener, a driver, two housemaids, and a cook. A bell was used to summon the domestic help, which seemed entirely normal for me and my siblings growing up. My parents' world, however, had completely transformed. Having travelled from north London to the Tropics, they were now enjoying what could be called a glamorous lifestyle, and the expectation was that they would simply adopt and adapt to these social privileges and unfamiliar social norms. And indeed they did, at least superficially. For example, throughout the 1950s, the communist party in Malaya fought a guerrilla war against the British, and one of our family stories is that my parents' car was accompanied by an armoured vehicle, allowing the family to gather safely with friends at the beach every weekend; nothing, not even a threat to their lives, was allowed get in the way of leisurely Sundays at the seaside.

Although British emergency rule had just about ended by the time I was born, I was brought up in an environment in which I was immersed in white social and economic advantage. My parents socialized with other white British, Irish, Australian, and European incomers. My two sisters, brother, and I lived with my parents in a large house on a hill overlooking the rubber plantation where my father employed and managed several hundred indigenous Malay, as well as Chinese and Indian, employees. Most were taken on as 'tappers', that is, they tapped the trees to harvest latex, which then becomes rubber. The plantation workers lived in what we called 'lines' on the estate. These were rows of hundreds of single-room, single-story, timber-stilted houses with basic facilities for sleeping, washing, and cooking. With repetition compulsion in mind, it has occurred to me that my father was commanding a labour camp within a war-torn country, of which he was now 'master'.

My siblings and I played with the children of our employees, spending time with them in the 'lines'. I remember close physical contact with our young maids (or amahs, as we called them) and they felt like family to me; our daily lives were enmeshed physically and emotionally with the local people, both adults and children. I remember sharing their food, spending time in their living quarters, lying on their beds. I have memories of our amahs dressing and playing with me and practising their make-up routines on me. My siblings and I were fluent in the Malay language as children – long forgotten now, unfortunately. As a child, I don't remember being aware of differences, let alone any family conversations taking place that referred to differences in status, levels of privilege, or skin colour, despite unequal power relationships being a defining feature of our home. Of course, this omission speaks to a denial of the racial and economic power dynamics that existed for colonial settlers at that time and in that context.

At eight years old I was sent to a boarding school in the UK. My older sisters and brother had already been dispatched to England. Here, we were educated alongside other children whose parents were also abroad enjoying the benefits of British colonialism. Because of the global distances between my own and my extended family members, there is a great deal of correspondence available for us to read now; letters exchanged between my mother and her parents in England, from my mother to us at school, and from us all to our parents, written during a period of over 20 years. Reading these letters since my mother and maternal grandmother's deaths has offered the opportunity for me to more clearly understand my mother's frame of mind as she settled abroad, and I've been particularly interested in reflecting on her experiences during the period of early motherhood.

Moving to a new country and leaving behind the familiar provokes a complex set of emotional responses. Of course, many migrant families have the necessary psychological resilience and thrive as a result of their choice to move across the world. However, my own mother's letters express many of the feelings that my young clients describe within their families, and which I see being played out, and unconsciously being responded to, in their lives. This is where I can see resonances with my own experiences of being parented. In my personal therapy I have also explored these memories and the impact my personal history has had on me.

Like many of my clients' parents, significant milestones and events during my parents' years abroad were not attended by members of their birth families. No one from my mother or father's families was present at my parents' wedding, for example, which took place at Penang Cathedral within a week of my mother's arrival in Malaya. Similarly, the births of each of my parents' four children happened without extended family on hand to support, encourage, or advise. My mother eventually made close friends in Malaya, but the absence of her own mother during this early period was evidently keenly felt. Starting a family without an extended family network can leave a new parent open to additional uncertainty and self-doubt. For example, there is an airmail letter exchange in which my mother anxiously asks my grandmother for advice about a minor illness my infant oldest sister is suffering, to which – because of the distance involved – she receives a reply several weeks later; too late, and once the panic is over. In her next letter, my mother apologizes profusely for worrying my grandmother and very soon stops asking for guidance about her young family, perhaps once she realizes that to do so caused my grandmother to worry and left her feeling helpless. At the same time, I hear in my mother's letters a desire to portray herself as a confident and capable mother to other planters' wives and, in many of her letters, I pick up on highly competitive feelings among the new mothers within my parents' social circle. The feelings of isolation and anxiety that may accompany new motherhood, compounded in my mother's case by the solitariness of rubber plantation life, seem to have been difficult to share. From her letters, I can hear that emotional support that might have been helpful was unavailable to, or not sought by, my mother in those early years.

From our practice as therapists, we are aware of the painful position that can come with feeling unable to express emotions for fear of impacting the 'loved object' while also feeling vulnerable to others' judgements. This may be the way a person feels when isolated in a new country. I'm conscious too that this way of relating can be picked up and echoed by children. My siblings and I spared our parents the worst of our distress on each occasion we left home to return to boarding school back in England. I have come to understand that we repressed our own feelings of loss and anguish in order to protect them from our pain and perhaps from their guilt, as well as to preserve an idealized image of them both. Like my clients' parents, my parents' choice to move country impacted deeply our experience of childhood. As Schaverien (2016) puts it in her description of what has become known as 'boarding school syndrome', the consequences of a wish to preserve the idealized image of the parent can be long-lasting and devastating for some:

> The child has to manage the bad feelings alone. In order to preserve the good image of the mother in her absence, the pain is experienced as a hated part of the self. This establishes a self-punishing, psychological splitting mechanism, which may continue into adulthood. (p. 22)

Within my family, my oldest sister took on aspects of the parenting role – stepping in as guardian when we were at school and during our travels back and forth to Malaysia. She often comforted me when I was distressed when away from home and, although her care was important to me, at the same time I felt her to be an inadequate substitute for my mother. My feelings of helplessness, terror, and confusion about being sent away were eventually rationalized as a way of defending against that agony. Schaverien describes this defence, often employed by boarding school children: "Whilst appearing to conform to the system, a form of unconscious splitting is acquired as a means of keeping the true self hidden" (Schaverien 2012: 141). Like many children who are sent away to school, it seems that my siblings and I gradually internalized the belief that what we understood to be our parents' needs – both making their life abroad and being protected from our distress – were more important than our own.

Through my practice and my own self-exploration, I am aware that when a child's basic need to express the whole spectrum of emotion and still feel loved becomes subordinated in order to accommodate parental needs, the child may then develop difficulties in expressing their authentic self (Winnicott, 1960/1990). In my work I listen to the stories of teenagers who moved to the UK with their families when they were children, leaving behind friends, grandparents, cousins, and even beloved pets. Sometimes my clients are able to describe how deeply shocked they felt by the move and their arrival in this country, often unable to speak English and initially feeling isolated and socially ostracized, particularly when they started school. I have never worked with a young person who is able to say that they felt psychologically prepared for their family's relocation to this country. My clients' sessions with me might be the first time that they have had the opportunity to explore and reflect on the loss, confusion, and helplessness they felt as a result of their parents' life-changing decision to migrate. I've found that clients can surprise themselves at the intensity of feeling these memories evoke.

Within my own family, children having been sent to boarding school meant that all 'loved objects' (except for my father) were out of my mother's reach for long periods of time. From my mother's letters to my grandparents, I'm aware that this situation was extraordinarily painful for both her and my father. As a result, we all unconsciously internalized the belief that expressing ambivalence within our family relationships was unacceptable. And here I mean between my siblings and myself as well as towards our parents. Time spent together during holidays was precious and voicing everyday discords and mixed feelings was discouraged. Minor conflicts that did occur have become woven into our family story and are occasions still referred to as exceptional, 50 years later. After migration, and when huge emotional losses have been experienced, great importance can be placed on holding the family group together: sibling relationships may become loaded with responsibility and significance; relationship fractures can become intolerable; and conflicting feelings within family relationships become difficult to own.

The reality, however, is that feelings about family members are always ambivalent and can be complex. For migrants, at the same time as family in the country of origin is missed, feelings of competitiveness may also arise and sometimes there may even be a desire (however unconscious) to 'triumph over' those left behind. Photographs sent back to the mother country often present a perfect image of life in the adopted country. The new life is portrayed as an unqualified success and there can be a desire to present an idealized account of the new way of living to those back 'home'. The adult migrants' reassurances to their own birth family may be the result of a combination of conscious and unconscious impulses: to vindicate the decision to have left, to protect the family of origin from worry, as well as a degree of competitiveness with the family that has been left behind. Moreover, there may be a desire to do the job of parenting perfectly (or perhaps better than their parents) as well as a wish to disavow aspects of their own family history or childhood story. Alongside the loss of a rooted identity is the possibility of re-inventing oneself and 'forgetting' shameful or guilty elements of family history completely. Tash Aw (2021), in his memoir *Strangers on a Pier*, which describes his family's experience of the East Asian diaspora from China via Malaysia to the UK, movingly explores the complexities of finding a sense of identity in a new country when rootedness and personal history have been left behind. He says: "All that is broken must remain in the past" (p.15).

At some level, whether consciously or unconsciously, the children of migrants are aware of the losses experienced and sacrifices made by their parents through moving to a new country. They frequently struggle with a felt sense of obligation to them. In our sessions, my clients explore their feelings of duty and desire to make their parents feel proud of their accomplishments, alongside feelings of responsibility and sometimes of open resentment about this obligation. Parents no longer have easy access to their family history and are making new lives without a grounded, contextualized sense of self. Feelings associated with 'child-contingent self-esteem' regularly emerge in the therapy (Kurz 2021). Kurz describes this as an "internalized concern for one's child's success", in which a parent hinges their own self-worth on their child's achievements (p. 10). According to Kurz, a combination of anxious and controlling child-rearing practices may be leading to an increase in perfectionism among young people in the western world (Ibid), which, combined with a fear of failure, is associated with high levels of anxiety and depression in children (Hewitt and Flett 1990; Sturman et al. 2009; Handley et al. 2014). In the general population, Speirs-Neumeister found that gifted young people whose self-worth is tied to achievement and a fear of disappointing others tend to be children who have experienced parental perfectionism and authoritarian parenting styles (Speirs-Neumeister 2004). In the context of migration, parents may focus on the need for their children to make the most of the opportunities available to them in the new country. This can sometimes lead to an anxious, critical, and controlling approach to parenting. Parents may unconsciously want their children to compensate for their own lack of opportunities of education or economic security, as well as make amends for their ongoing feelings of loss and emotional privation. They may feel that it is their family group's duty to the ancestors and wider family to make a success of the move abroad. This felt pressure, together with a fragile sense of self and a hypersensitivity to failure, can mean that parents demand that their children achieve the highest levels of academic success: "The future is lived vicariously through their [children's] achievements: their lives must follow an upward trajectory. They must not fail" (Aw 2021: 90).

Among young people of any background, complex feelings about the pressure to succeed can lead to self-sabotage by procrastinating or 'downing tools' – an unconscious and self-directed rebellion against giving their parents the success they feel is being demanded of them. These difficult-to-acknowledge feelings can be underpinned by a deeper sense of not feeling heard and of being misunderstood; young people in therapy regularly comment that their parents can't possibly understand the academic pressure they are experiencing, given that they haven't been through the same education system themselves.

Together with the concern that they, and their children, should make the most of what is available in the new country, parents can have a strong sense of missing out on what they have left behind. The country of origin can become idealized and comes to symbolize all that is good. In the therapy room, I hear an unconscious 'splitting' taking place for some of the parents of the young people I work with: the 'mother' country is described to their children as an idyllic place, which provided an untroubled, simple, and carefree existence. Of course, for many of my clients' parents the country they came from is where they themselves were children, and therefore these may be true depictions of parts of their own childhoods. For my clients' parents, in Klein's terms, the country of origin has come to symbolize 'the good breast' (Klein 1946), while the adopted country signifies its opposite – all that is harsh and difficult about adulthood. The young people I work with sometimes align with their parents in this view, idealizing the country that has been left behind, or, alternatively, for some, that place becomes a locus for condemning their parents – the country where their parents originated from may be described as 'backward', 'ignorant', and 'brutal'. This can be understood as an unconscious symbolic attack – criticizing the 'mother' country becomes a derogation of the parent.

My own experiences of parental migration and, perhaps equally importantly, subsequent separations from my parents, have made a deeply affecting impact on my sense of self and belonging. About ten years ago my husband, daughter, and I travelled to Malaysia. For me it was the first time since my family had left the country. In many ways it was the trip of a lifetime and I was curious to see how it would feel for me to return there, especially as it had taken me a very long time to decide to go back. A part of me hoped for and expected a flood of warm memories, aroused by familiar smells, scenes, places, and tastes evoking the loving early childhood I had experienced. Sadly, I didn't feel at home at all. In the event, nothing I found there matched up to the idealized image of childhood I had been holding on to and, in fact, I found that during some parts of the holiday I felt unaccountably anxious. This felt to me like an echo of aspects of my mother's experiences, and therefore perhaps elements of my own as a child. When we visited the houses, towns, and beaches I had spent time in until the age of 11, it wasn't easy; I felt unsettled and out of sorts. Even the Malay food we ate there, which I find delicious here at home, and which has been familiar to me from birth, felt 'other' and didn't offer any Proustian comfort.

I enjoyed the scenery, our jungle walks, the wildlife, and the spectacular beaches, just as any holidaymaker would, but I really didn't feel like I belonged.

Clinical material and some personal reflections

In the final section of this chapter, I consider the material of a client I worked with some years ago in a mainstream secondary school's Sixth Form whose story of family relocation evoked moments of recognition for me. Some details have been altered to protect her anonymity.

Uzma, in her final year at school when we met, was referred for therapy because she'd been experiencing panic attacks. Her parents had moved to London from South Asia when she was four years old. Her mother was in her late twenties when they arrived in the UK to join an uncle here on Uzma's father's side of the family. Uzma now had an older sister of 23 and a younger sibling who was born in the UK.

Uzma described herself as 'unemotional', saying she had a tendency to 'dissociate'. She told me she had self-injured in the past, using a pin to scratch at her arm. Uzma said she's 'always been a perfectionist' and was now puzzled by why her 'low-level stress' had begun manifesting as panic attacks, which were getting in the way of her studies. She was demure and neatly presented with a clear open face and sat on the front edge of her seat as she talked in a quiet voice. Uzma tells me that, because of her overwhelming feelings of panic, she has decided to postpone her application to university to study medicine and plans to take a gap year. This is not being well received by her wider family, some of whom now live in the UK, but who she feels have little understanding of the education system and of her emotional needs. At the same time as she is frustrated by her family's lack of knowledge about the English education system, she also worries that she will disappoint them. She says this feeling of letting them down is adding to her anxiety, as she would very much like to make her parents proud of her achievements.

Uzma tells me that she attended one of the other local secondary schools until Year 10 when she transferred to this school, as her parents didn't feel that the academic standards at her first school were good enough; "But I've always got them the grades", she says. She describes how the wish to become a doctor is long-standing and entirely her own and that her mother just wants her to be happy; the idea of Uzma letting her mother know of her distress would be unthinkable. Uzma describes her mother as warm and loving, telling me about the sacrifices her mother has made for the family, how hard her mother works, and how she has never seen her mother cry. Uzma's father drives a taxi for a living and she rarely sees him. She spends time in her room and she says her dad's usually either busy at work or on his phone. Uzma's father is the oldest in his birth family and Uzma knows that he regularly sends money home to his parents in their country of origin. Uzma tells me she feels fortunate to no longer live in the country of her birth: "I feel like if we'd stayed, I might just have ended up as a village girl", she says with some contempt. Uzma has a complex relationship with her older sister who, being six years older, did much of the childcare when they were growing up. Uzma resents this and has a fractious relationship with this sister while she feels a real alignment with her younger brother for whom she intends to be a role model. Uzma's sister went to university but dropped out at the end of the first year and is back living in the family home. All of Uzma's fury is directed towards her sister; she tells me that her sister treated her cruelly when she was responsible for her care while their parents were at work. Uzma says that she feels her mother favours her sister and I have the strong sense that Uzma has missed out on a full relationship with both her mum and dad. The competition between Uzma and her sister is fierce and Uzma's fervent wish is to triumph over her sister in her studies. Uzma's mother, while portrayed as gentle and loving, continues to be less emotionally available than Uzma would like.

The therapy with Uzma offered an opportunity to explore the family's experiences in relational as well as psychoanalytic terms. She and I thought together about how, out of necessity, family members had missed out on various roles and opportunities they might have expected – her older sister becoming responsible for caring while still a child herself, as their parents became preoccupied with earning a living for the family shortly after their arrival in this country. We wondered together if her older sister had enacted her anger about the move to this country by bullying Uzma. We explored Uzma's feelings about leaving her country of birth and the beloved grandmother they left behind. We thought about the motivation for her decision to train as a doctor and the tremendous fear this evokes in her as the responsibilities and reality of this future come into view. In our sessions, working with a family map, Uzma considered the possible relationship to their home country from each family member's perspective and how the move here might have been experienced for them. And, what of Uzma's relationship with her mother who, together with Uzma's father, initiated the relocation? What about Uzma's feelings of ambivalence in this relationship? Early on in the therapy, expressing any mixed emotions towards her mother seemed impossible: "Mum's done everything for me and she's one of my best friends". Uzma then began to wonder if her panic attacks were related to her inability to share her concerns about the future and feelings about past losses with her parents. Gradually, as Uzma began to explore her own relationship with each of her family members in depth, she began to reflect on the possibility that her sister may be carrying her own set of unexplored feelings about the move to this country. Uzma started to acknowledge the complexity of the whole family's experience of relocating and assimilating. She wondered if her mum's perceived favouritism of her sister might be related to her mum's guilty feelings about extracting the family from their roots. Uzma began to reflect on how the extreme pressure she feels to achieve might be built on complex emotional reactions to the life changes and losses experienced by the whole family.

The details of Uzma's family migration story differ from my own in many ways. But despite these material differences, elements of the migrant experience are common to us both and there are relational aspects within our families which echo each other as well. Seeing me as a white, middle-aged woman, Uzma could never know that her life story features processes and emotions that resonate so deeply with my own. Nor did I ever tell her. I can only hope that through my efforts to really listen, the working relationship we developed over time and my unconscious communications within the therapy setting, Uzma felt that I fully understood important elements of her life experience. For myself, and perhaps for Uzma too, therapy has offered an experience through which

> we see our parents or siblings … with their *own* inadequacies…. We examine at a feeling level the parental introjects, and in so doing, we come to have an experience inside ourselves of their perspective … We experience ourselves in relation to differing subjectivities and the way in which we are affected by and affect the other.
>
> (Orbach 2014: 23–24)

One aim of the work with Uzma was to offer her routes to exploring and expressing the whole range of her emotional response to her life-shaping early experiences. In turn, working with Uzma afforded me an opportunity to reflect once again on aspects of my own life processes, including my family's experiences of assimilation, the roots of my own feelings around dislocation and belonging, my personal history of separation and loss, as well as offering another reminder that the search for inner ease can feel like a daring adventure in itself.

References

Aw, T. (2021) *Strangers on a Pier: Portrait of a Family*, London: Fourth Estate.

Freud, S. (1961) *Beyond the Pleasure Principle* (O. Strachey, ed. and trans.). New York, NY: W. W. Norton. (Original work published 1920).

Handley, A.K., Egan, S.J., Kane, R.T. et al. (2014) 'The relationships between perfectionism, pathological worry and generalised anxiety disorder', *BMC Psychiatry* 14: 98. https://doi.org/10.1186/1471-244X-14-98

Hewitt, P.L. and Flett, G.L. (1990) 'Perfectionism and depression: A multidimentional analysis', *Journal of Social Behaviour and Personality* 5(5): 423.

Klein, M. (1946) 'Notes on some schizoid mechanisms', *International Journal of Psycho-Analysis* 27: 99–110.

Kurz, E. (2021) 'The rise of perfectionism', *European Journal of Psychotherapy and Counselling* 23(1): 1–14.

Orbach, S. (2014) 'I wanted the stuff of secrets to be in the light', in S. Kuchuck (ed.) *Clinical Implications of the Psychoanalyst's Life Experience*. London: Routledge: 17–25.

Schaverien, J. (2012) 'Boarding school syndrome: Broken Attachments, a hidden trauma', *British Journal of Psychotherapy* 28(3): 138–155.

Schaverien, J. (2016) 'Exiled: The girls' school boarders', *Therapy Today* 27(9): 20–23.

Speirs-Neumeister, K.L. (2004) 'Factors influencing development of perfectionism in gifted college students', *Gifted Child Quarterly* 48(4): 259.

Sturman, E.D., Flett, G.L., Hewitt, P.L. and Rudolph, S.G. (2009) 'Dimensions of perfectionism and self-worth contingencies in depression', *Journal of Rational-Emotive & Cognitive Behavior Therapy* 27: 213–231.

Winnicott, D.W. (ed.) (1990) 'Ego distortion in terms of true and false self', *The Maturational Process and the Facilitating Environment: Studies in the Theory of Emotional Development*. London: Karnac: 140–152. (Original work published 1960.)

Chapter 5

Mother and other tongues
Personal experiences and clinical reflections

Stefania Putzu-Williams

In psychoanalytic thinking, the mother's voice is understood to have an important containing function for the infant. The tone, pitch, and cadence 'wrap' the baby in a cocoon of words, the meaning of which is conveyed through sound alone (Segal 1957; Anzieu 1976). As the attachment bond strengthens and the infant starts to integrate his perception of the mother, they also begin to organise sounds: babbling changes into words and words acquire a magic value, for it is with words that the child reaches out across the gap to connect with the mother[1].

Words also recreate what might seem to have been lost. When there is good enough attunement, the child experiences his vocalising or words as eliciting a response from the mother. As time unfolds, the internal world of the child is slowly built from the foundations laid by this emotionally invested earliest form of 'to and fro' communication. Thus, our mother tongue is our archaic heritage, as it carries within a view of the world rooted in all the childhood experiences, memories, and feelings dating back to the beginning of life. But what if there are two maternal figures and two mother tongues? How might this affect the baby's 'felt experience' and shape their inner landscape?

I was born in Cagliari, the capital of Sardinia, in Italy, a city of circa 300,000 habitants on the seaside on the south coast of Sardinia. I studied Psychology at Rome University, La Sapienza, where I met my future husband at 24 and moved to England two years later; I married 'a real Englishman', we used to joke. After marriage, we moved to the UK in 1985 where we lived in Folkestone and Bournemouth for a couple of years, still by the sea, but cold, and then in London for the past 37 years. I am a psychologist, and a supervisor, and work full-time as a psychodynamic counsellor based in two inner London multicultural and multilingual secondary academies. I work with clients and I had my personal therapy in what is for me a second language acquired in adulthood. My interest in language usage in psychotherapy, and in particular the subject of bilingualism, was stimulated by my work in schools with young people who spoke more than one language, or who didn't speak their mother tongue, and by the personal experience of therapy when I came into contact, through the transference relationship, with early memories around being brought up in a

DOI: 10.4324/9781003270447-6

family of professional Italian parents and a live-in nanny we called 'Tata' (who, lived in our family home for 29 years, moving out, coincidentally, when I got married and left the country).

As an infant, Tata spoke and sang to me in Sardo, Sardinian, her mother tongue, although she was also fluent in Italian, the language we spoke in the family. Tata mainly spoke Sardinian with my maternal grandmother. Sardinians have their own language, a neo-Latin/Romance language, with its own dictionary, grammar, and usage and different dialects are spoken regionally within the island. Italian became the official language of Sardinia in 1760 but only became widespread after the last world war, with the beginning of compulsory education. Sardinians could be defined as 'native' bilinguals, even though their original language is less and less commonly spoken by new generations; while Italian is generally considered more sophisticated and the language of the educated (or, one could say, of the coloniser), speaking Sardinian can have a more negative connotation, often denoting inferiority, ignorance, and associated with a lower, or so-called 'peasant' class. Feelings of shame and ridicule used to surround speaking Sardinian, commonly used to humour, mock, and joke, so that although many understand Sardinian, most do not actually speak it. It was only in the 1970s and 80s that a movement began to press for the revaluation of the culture, music, language, and history of Sardinia, which archaeology dates as 3,500ac years old. However, currently Sardinia history and language are still not studied or spoken in schools.

During my MSc degree course in psychodynamic counselling and psychotherapy, now some time ago, reading the literature on bilingualism and having therapy in my newly acquired language, made me reflect on the meaning of my experience of having 'two mothers' and two mother tongues from infanthood. I realised I had a 'forgotten' language, Sardo. I came to see how early experiences were being replayed in my later life and in therapy in the transference. It made me think about the emotional investment, the many unconscious expectations and motivations in marrying an Englishman, moving to a foreign country, learning a new language, studying and training in a new language, and choosing to bring up bilingual and 'bi/multicultural' children. I slowly began to realise the degree to which my choices had been partly guided by internal demands. However, I learned that this kind of 'maternal split' is only healed when it is owned and the feelings evoked, understood. The learning of a new language, English, also made me realise how relative and arbitrary are the ways in which our own language describes the world, and I became more aware of the value judgements invoked by certain words and forms of expression. 'Politically correct' terminology is the most obvious example of these phenomena.

At the first encounter with the new language, English, the sound of the foreign words sometimes gave me, particularly, when tired and sleepy, a feeling of comfort, of a place where I could retreat to a sort of 'reverie' in which I felt held by the sound of different accents and inflections and by words I did not yet understand. I suppose the sound of words felt like a comforting lullaby.

At other times, the sound of the English words felt intolerably 'foreign', harsh, and meaningless. The lack of understanding of the foreign language and difficulty expressing myself in this new language, reactivated feelings of being de-skilled and infantilised, and I felt frustrated. For some time I was unable to verbally express abstract or theoretical reasoning and spontaneous expression was a challenge when I was still in the process of translating from Italian to English. The impossibility of making or understanding jokes, of playing with words and, ultimately, being myself, felt like a loss of a sense of identity. Our perception, and the sense we make of the world around us, is both arrived at and articulated through language; therefore language is indissolubly woven into the fabric of the self.

After many decades of living in London and regularly going back to Italy twice a year, I now feel I have two home countries. The fluent use and 'switch' between languages is something I take for granted. I am aware, for example, that when interacting with different people I find I use a different language depending on the situation and emotional contact. We know for instance, that a concept is more easily accessible in the language in which it was learned. I feel I have arrived at a settled place which allows for an ease of flow between languages and expressions. The learning of a new language and the experience of therapy allowed for old conflicts to be thought about and spoken in new words. Also, going back and forth between languages (and countries) perhaps implies some hope of bridging a gap: the original split and the sensation of being 'in between' cultures, languages, and 'mothers', perhaps compelled me to 'get more of the same' in an unconscious search to reunite and seek integration.

Language is always acquired in a relational context, originally within the mother/child dyad. What is being shaped between mother and child are not only words but also meanings and new relationships with the world. In parallel with learning to talk, the small child is getting used to the experience of being separate from the mother and the loss of intimacy this implies. Words and 'ways of being' keep the mother alive in the child's mind as well as making it possible to distinguish between 'me' and 'not me' (Winnicott 1965). In psychoanalytic psychotherapy, words can be used for the expression and resolution of infantile conflicts, including those dating from before the client's acquisition of speech. However, researchers in the field report that the use of a second language offers bilingual clients the opportunity to build up a defensive system against their infantile life. Costa (2020) found that traumatised clients, notably refugees, may feel overwhelmed to speak in the language in which the trauma was experienced and the newly acquired language works as a 'barrier' against traumatic experiences and painful feelings linked to childhood of loss and attachment. At other times there is a need for the client to tell their story in their mother tongue or another language, for example with bereavement, and the therapist allows this by inviting the client to then translate it for them. The cognitive action of translation can decode and decrease the intensity of the traumatic event, facilitating the emotional response and communication.

As I have noted in reference to my own experiences, this is because a second language may never be emotionally invested in the same way as the mother tongue. There is a detachment, a distancing. In her autobiography Eva Hoffman (1989:106) gives a vivid sense of the power of words and what some words evoke in us:

> The words I learn now don't stand for things in the same unquestioned way they did in my native tongue. "River" in Polish was a vital sound, energized with the essence of riverhood, of my rivers, of my being immersed in rivers. "River" in English is cold – a word without an aura. It has no accumulated associations for me, and it does not give off the radiating haze of connotation. It does not evoke.

Regarding bilingual and multilingual individuals, some questions arise about the close relationship between mother and mother tongue: for example, what happens when more than one language is spoken from the beginning to the infant – and what are the implications if these different languages are spoken by the same person, for example, the mother, or another carer (as in my personal experience). Also, how is it internally represented, that is, can these two aspects be separated, or do they form part of the whole relationship with the maternal image? In the case of international adoptions, for example, what happens at an unconscious level when the mother tongue is abandoned and becomes silent and the new language replaces it completely?

Reflecting on how a second language can be infused with deeper emotional resonance when it is used within a mother/child relationship or family constellation, I have noticed, for example, how my relationship with the English language is ever evolving and speaking both languages with my own children has certainly enriched it for me. Speaking Italian with my children and reading bedtime stories in Sardinian suggests the conscious and unconscious wish to connect with both my native languages and with my two mothers, creating an intimate 'maternally defined space' with my children. The father can feel excluded, as the children become 'native speakers' like the mother. However,

> every child will experience a series of exiles … As the child turns away from the mother's body towards the language of the father, moving from the imaginary to the symbolic realm, there begins the process of naming things and using language and the environment.
>
> (John Clare 2004:12)

Perhaps even if the father can speak the language, as in my case, it might never create the same emotionally invested experience as that which the mother has with her children to whom she has spoken her mother tongue from infancy onwards. However, when the languages spoken are interwoven in the family interactions and shared, the usage of more languages allows integration and inclusion, rather than splitting and guilt-inducing feelings about excluding or 'erasing' the father. 'It requires the sensitivity and openness to linguistic difference' or as Costa calls it, 'linguistic empathy' (Costa 2020:12).

Turning to my practice as a school-based psychotherapist, I can see how the students I work with who are using an acquired language face an added complexity in navigating the already vertiginous and often confusing adolescent years. In the midst of their fluid identities and process of self-discovery (or at times dread and avoidance of self-knowledge), a new language, a new country and culture, often a new family set up, can be very difficult to adjust to. The pulls between who we are and who we are becoming, the sense of self, the feeling of belonging, the lack of emotional attachment, all create tensions and challenges needing new adjustments.

However, Cederic Bouet-Willaumez (2021) suggests that "a new language is a new representation of mother" (2021:77–93) and quoting theories from Greenson and Stengel, "It seemed that in learning a new language, we create a new inner representation of our mother, which coexists with the one that was formed earlier". Velikowski believes that "a recently acquired language could become a language of the unconscious" (Amati-Mehler, Argentieri, & Canestri 1944). The new language and the mother tongue are like a 'transitional space' between languages and cultures.

The experience of acquiring a new language can also be rewarding as I have found personally and in the lives of some of the students I have worked with. A new identity can be formed around the second language which can bring the pleasures and challenges of engaging in new roles in a different setting and new context, as was the case with Carla, a student I saw for just over three years.

Carla was a 15-year-old Italian girl who moved to London in the summer and joined the school in September. She did not speak English, although she had studied it at school in Italy. She was the older child in the family, initially left behind with her grandmother in Italy when her parents moved to London following their young son's death at 4. Her parents eventually settled in the UK with Father securing work while Mother stayed at home and managed the family's finances. They later had two young daughters who were aged 4 and 3 when Carla joined them.

Carla spent her formative years in Italy and was brought up by her grandmother and grandfather. She went to school in the nearest city to their village where she made some friends. On arriving in London when she was 15, everything was new for her: she had two young sisters and what felt like new parents. After eight years spent living apart, she felt no meaningful connection with her mother and father and the separation from her grandmother was experienced as a significant loss. When I met her, Carla was in a new country, a new school and speaking a new language, and adapting to a new environment.

A teacher specialising in English as an additional language (EAL) referred Carla for counselling in school because Carla, worried and frightened, had confided in her that, at times, she felt like killing herself, especially when her mother made what Carla perceived as critical remarks about her. I learned that Carla spoke very little English and was therefore pushed back a year making her the oldest amongst her peers. In the counselling sessions, we established a good relationship, helped, no doubt by the two of us speaking mainly in Italian for the first phase of our work about Carla's sense of being an outsider within her family and among her peer group, and missing her grandmother, her home country, and her old school friends, and feeling at a loss loss with social cues; these were all common themes.

Carla spoke about her childhood memories in Italian. She initially struggled with her peer group in school, feeling out of step with their norms and interests. In particular, she could not understand why her classmates stood so close together and touched, kissed, and hugged each other so frequently. This opened up talk of her childhood, where contrary to the Italian stereotype, Carla had no memories of any kind of physical contact with her parents before they left for London or since re-joining them more recently. It may be that her brother's death, and her parents' withdrawal through grief, threw into sharp relief a more general lack of physical comfort and warmth in the family. It was possible that Carla's arrival in London reminded her mother of the painful loss of her son.

Carla became increasingly fluent in English, her confidence grew and she began to make good progress in school. A new language seemed to have given Carla a new lease on life as it provided a fresh way of looking at and seeing herself, whilst I witnessed her story unfolding. As the therapy progressed, the learning of the new language allowed Carla to tell her story using both Italian and English, exploring her relationships, her friendships, and her new experiences in London. I listened carefully, and at times 'performed' as her memory by linking events, noticing patterns when speaking in the different languages, and looking at their meaning. It was fascinating to witness the switch between languages and how frequently memories of childhood were spoken in her mother tongue, often with fondness but also with some critical undertones, while contemporary issues and stories were recounted in English in a newly-discovered 'chatty adolescent'. This dynamic can be seen as part of the affective detachment found in bilingual individuals which can be 'protective' and helpful by weakening the strength of the superego, when the superego that corresponds to the first language is overcritical and harsh or when trauma has been experienced.

Various studies on bilingual adults, observations by clinicians, researchers in the field of psychoanalysis, as well as in the work of many creative writers, suggest agreement that speaking in a foreign language, in particular a later second language acquisition, produces affective detachment in the bilingual individual.

I worked with Carla for just over three years. She was able to use therapy well and switch thoughtfully between the two languages, the language of childhood and the new language, including the 'adolescent' language with slang and various mannerisms, identity, and a different vision of the world. I became for Carla a new kind of attachment figure and was able to function as a secure base for her, a process greatly helped by sharing a mother tongue with her. When she left the Sixth Form for university, she kept in touch with me via my work email. I learned that she recently married a young Italian man and is doing very well. It seems reasonable to assume that our coming together as a therapeutic couple was fortuitous, perhaps for both of us. Although the work was at times challenging as it put me in close touch with my own history of migration and all that this entailed, including feeling like an outsider, these experiences gave me an internal map that perhaps Carla sensed.

It is a relief for young people such as Carla to learn that none of us are defined solely by one aspect of our personality, and that we all need to be able to tolerate and enjoy our many sides. Everyone has different ways of relating, different self-states, affective moods, as well as patterns of thinking, conflicting feelings and ambivalence, and sometimes different languages too. We learn about ourselves, develop new skills, and perform new roles in our lives by seeing how we are perceived by others as well as hearing about their lives and how they understand the world. A sense of self and one's own identity develops and evolves through these relational exchanges and encounters, each bringing the possibility of new and transformative experiences.

Many young people find counselling helps them to better use their native tongue or acquired language, alongside social skills, friendships, subcultures, and reflections on identity to 'bridge the gaps', ensuring they can make meaningful connections and form mutually fulfilling relationships with peers and with the adults in their lives. Often, this comes about through speaking freely and playing with ideas. This can be more difficult to achieve at first if a client is speaking English as an additional language. However even in such cases, as the relationship with the therapist develops, and the young person acclimatises to the way therapy works, creating a common language, generally, a 'loosening up' occurs which allows for greater fluency and an increase in free association. The possibility of verbalising experiences in the language in which they occurred can be transformative, enabling the expression of early memories, primary experiences, and bodily sensations with emotional resonance.

If there is a lack of a sufficient knowledge of the language(s) including the idioms or 'slang' used in therapy, the therapist and client might be more likely to find they do not share the same associations to words. My own therapy brought to light how the meaning of emotionally charged experiences can be lost in translation at least while the acquired language is still a relatively new one. Also, I saw how a word or phrase used by the therapist evoked a feeling or affective memory in me that at times was very different from that to which the therapist was referring. Still, these obstacles can be transformed into opportunities to enrich communication if both therapist and client are willing to find new ways to express themselves and find a shared meaning.

When we change languages, both our world view and our identities get transformed. We need to become new selves to speak a language that does not come from our core self, a language that does not reflect our inner-connectedness with the culture it represents (Imberti 2007:71). We build our sense of self, not just through the words we use to describe ourselves to ourselves but also through the meaning we give to the language we speak and the accent we may have. My two 'birth languages' – Italian and Sardinian – each evoke particular sets of values, associations, and related affect. In common with many, I was brought up to view the Italian language as 'superior' and Sardinian as 'inferior', even shame-inducing. Regrettably, ranking languages and accents as 'better than' or 'less than' continues to feature in contemporary culture despite the pushback against such forms of discrimination and prejudice. More optimistically, language never stands still and young people find their own way to step outside of some of the more unhelpful frames of reference. Some rap music and poetry performed as 'spoken word' provide opportunities to share and collectively process experiences while also conveying more uplifting messages. There will always be a place for therapy, too: most young people intuitively respond to the kind of attentive listening therapists provide, despite the differences in age, race, culture, and even language. Although I was able to speak to Carla in her 'mother tongue', the 'felt experience' of being in a very particular kind of space together and our mutual attempts to understand and relate to each other often transcended language itself.

The close relationship between 'mother' and 'mother tongue' including what happens when more than one language is spoken to the infant from the beginning, makes me think about how some people maintain the accent from the mother tongue in the new language, which could be seen as a way of sustaining one's own sense of identity and perhaps reflects an unconscious sense of guilt for one's own betrayal (that is, the betrayal of abandoning the 'mother tongue'). Kristeva calls the suffering involved in giving up the birth language as 'a sort of matricide' (Julia Kristeva 2000:166). While vocabulary and grammar have to be learned, the accent, intonation, and rhythm of speech are incorporated through imitation.

Beverley Costa (2020) set up a counselling service in Reading, called Mothertongue, offering culturally and linguistic sensitive counselling and therapy to local black and ethnic communities. She underlines in her book *Other Tongues* how multilingual people are different from monolingual people. "In the multilingual client, the nature of emotion(s) or feeling(s) they wish to talk about and understand in the course of therapy may require them to switch languages". The therapist needs to allow this, by asking the client, when suitable or if there is an impasse, to speak their chosen language, then translate it into English for the therapist. Costa talks about 'Linguistic empathy' (Costa 2020: 12) as an openness to linguistic differences, inviting the client to tell the story in their own language, which is not spoken by the therapist, and then the client 'back-translates' it into English so that the therapist can understand. By doing this "the cognitive act of translating it into English helps the client to find a different, more empowered position in relation to the words" (ibid: 15).

Conclusion

This chapter has hopefully provided an overview of some of the issues relating to language usage in psychotherapy and the relationships between 'mother' and 'mother tongue' and early language development. Reflecting on my own experience, I attempted to explore how the different languages may be internally represented in the bilingual individual and considered some aspects of the relationship between language, culture, and sense of identity. The usage of more than one language in psychotherapy produces many interesting theoretical and technical queries. The research found that most people feel different when they use different languages therefore their behaviour will be also different (Dawaele 2016).

The phenomenon of emotional detachment associated with speaking a second language and exploration of the advantages and disadvantages and meaning of using more than one language in therapy, particularly stimulated my interest. They generated many thoughts about my personal and professional experience, including my role as a 'foreign' psychologist who trained as a psychodynamic counsellor in my newly acquired language, and undertook psychotherapy in the new language. I illustrated working in therapy in two languages – the mother tongue, and the newly acquired second language for the client – with a clinical vignette of 'Carla' who represents a composite of students I have seen over many years in my school-based practice. Switching between languages and choice of language in therapy revealed aspects of my young client's personality in relation to the language used and its internal representations. Although sharing the same languages in therapy is no guarantee of a successful outcome, and the emphasis is rather on the therapeutic relationship itself, when the psychotherapist matches the patient's languages, by working along with the languages, incorporating and using them, it appears to add a useful dimension and richness to the psychotherapeutic intervention.

Note

1 In her work on symbol formation Segal (1957) describes the development from early symbols, which are hardly different from the original object and also from the self, called 'symbolic equations', from the fully formed symbols in the depressive position. The awareness of differentiation and separateness between the ego and the object, the now fully experienced ambivalence, and the concern for saving the object from his aggression and possessiveness, "is a powerful stimulus for the creation of symbols" (394) which *are* used to overcome loss rather than deny it. One of the tasks of the ego in the depressive position is to lessen anxieties and resolve conflicts not only of the depressive kind, but also to deal with earlier unresolved

conflicts by symbolising them. Segal also affirms that symbols are needed not only to communicate with the external world, but also in the internal communication with one's unconscious and oneself, and believes that this capacity to communicate with oneself by means of symbols – words as the basis of verbal thinking. Segal concludes saying:

> The word 'symbol' comes from the Greek term ... bringing together, integrating. The process of symbol formation is, I think, a continuous process of bringing together and integrating the internal with the external, the subject with the object, and the earlier experiences with the later ones. (397)

References

Amati-Mehler, J, Argentieri, S, & Canestri, J (1994) *The Babel of the Unconscious*, Madison, CT: International Universities Press.

Anzieu, D (1976) Narciso. *La envoltura Sonora del si mismo*. Novelle Revue de Psychanalyse 13. Quoted in Grinberg & Grinberg (1989).

Bouet-Willaumez, C (2021) Silence, dissonance, and harmony: Integrating the multilingual self. (77–93). In: *Mother Tongue and Other Tongues. Narratives in Multilingual Psychotherapy*. Ed. Ali Zarbifi and Shulka Wilson. Phoenix Publishing House Bicester, Oxfordshire.

Clare, J (2004) *Introduction to Lost Childhood and the Language of Exile*. Ed. Judith Szekacs-Weisz & Ivan Ward, London: Imago East West; Freud Museum.

Costa, B. (2020) *Other Tongues. Psychological Therapies in a Multilingual World*, Monmouth: PCCS Books.

Dawaele, J-M (2016) Why so many bi- and multilingual feel different when switching languages? *International Journal of Multilingualism* 13:92–105.

Hoffman, E (1998) *Lost in Translation*, London: Vintage.

Imberti, P (2007) Who resides behind the words? Exploring and understanding the language experience of the non-English-speaking immigrant. *Family in Society: The Journal of Contemporary Social Services* 88(1):67–73.

Kristeva, J (2000) *"Bulgaria my Suffering"* in Crisis of the European Subject. New York: Other Press.

Segal, H (1957) Notes on symbol formation. *Integrated Journal of Psychology Analysis* 38:391–397.

Winnicott, DW (1965) *The Maturational Process and the Facilitating Environment: Studies in the Theory of Emotional Development*. London: Tavistock.

Chapter 6

The Biafran War

A transgenerational legacy

Angela Ike

If a movie were ever made about my mother's life, the inciting incident would be the Biafran war and the loss of my maternal grandfather. I say loss rather than death because having gone missing he became quite literally lost. After several decades he was accepted as dead and because Igbo people (in my opinion) are astute about life's processes, when my grandmother died, my mother and her siblings dug two graves in my grandfather's compound. So as a nine-year-old, I attended the burial of both my maternal grandparents within days of one another.

After my grandmother's interment, a symbolic burial was held for my grandfather with a coffin containing soil from the place where he was believed to have been last sighted. This was done so that his children and extended family could have a formal opportunity to mourn and a reference point for their grief. When I think of this event, I am often reminded of the saying "dust to dust, ashes to ashes" and its aptness here.

The Biafran War, a Nigerian Civil War occurring between mid-1967 and early 1970 was a civil war between Nigeria and the breakout nation of Biafra during which many Biafran (mainly Igbo) people were killed and many more were forced to flee to their home villages in South Eastern Nigeria carrying whatever they could of their possessions on their person. Horror stories abound from my parents, extended family members, and literature about the time of pregnant women being stabbed in the stomach, air raid attacks on villages, orphaned children, Kwashiorkor victims, and abject poverty, some of which was experienced by my mother, her siblings, and my grandmother.

For my mother this occurred at a crucial developmental stage in her life as a young teenager coming of age and (according to her) entering that phase where she felt she could start to engage in banter with her parents. My mother described many times throughout her life one of the last conversations she had with her father when they were walking to school and work respectively one morning. She relayed him teasing her about always wearing the same cardigan, her teasing him back about his mac and the two of them sharing a laugh. My mother clearly loved my grandfather who she described as a kind, gentle, and wise man whom she felt she was just getting to know beyond the strict bounds

DOI: 10.4324/9781003270447-7

of a father–daughter relationship when he was lost to the family. My mother would mourn the loss of her father for the rest of her life.

As a result of my mother's mourning I too have always mourned my grandfather. In actuality, I lost both my grandfathers to the Biafran war and although my father was older (in his twenties) with a different story to tell (he was studying in Britain at the time and joined the various protests about the war) and has rarely spoken about his loss, as I have come to see it, the impact has manifested itself in various ways in his life.

The Biafran war created a multigenerational layer of mourning from my grandmothers to my parents and cousins and I that is both unique to our families and us as individuals. As Kyle Ikeda very aptly states in his book *Okinawan War Memory* "although second generation survivors may not be direct victims of violent or traumatic events, they are witnesses to the effects of war and trauma on the lives of their parents" (Ikeda, 2017: 33). I would take this one step further and say that in witnessing the impact of war and trauma on our parents, as second-generation survivors we not only share their loss, distress, and sense of disempowerment about the events that occurred, we can often have an added layer of distress of our own. This at least in my experience comes from witnessing those we love continuing to grapple with the effect of their trauma and noticing the way in which it impacts their sense of self and their interactions with the world. Observing one's parent be both simultaneously incredibly capable and severely wounded is awe-inspiring but also unspeakably sad. I think the legacy of the Biafran war on me as a second-generation war survivor is one of a latent sorrow that I have lived with my entire life. For my part, I have and always will long for the grandfathers I never knew because their lives were invariably cut short and I have had to navigate my sadness and anger about this my entire life. I have also always had a sense of the precariousness of life and the world as a potentially rapidly changeable place. As Jung (1968) aptly put it in his seminal work *The Archetypes and the Collective Unconscious* "the collective unconscious does not develop individually but is inherited. It consists of pre-existent forms…. which can only become conscious secondarily and which give definite form in certain psychic contents" (p. 43).

So how does this translate to my work? Well firstly, it is no coincidence I am a therapist or that I was a journalist before that. On the face of it, these professions may seem far removed from one another but when you look closely you see that they are both fundamentally about providing people with the opportunity to tell their stories, documenting these accounts, and acknowledging their validity. In other words, bearing witness. As a therapist I see one of the fundamental functions of my role as simply being there to listen and walk alongside the client as they narrate and attempt to make sense of their trajectory, whilst acknowledging that I hear and see them. This alone can be so powerful with often very little need for any other form of intervention.

I was always bound to be interested in transgenerational trauma. It would be a denial and disconnection from myself and my history to be otherwise. The fact that I chose to train as a psychodynamic counsellor, a discipline that concerns itself with how the past influences current feelings, thinking, and behaviour, is no great surprise to me either. When contemplating becoming a therapist, I availed myself of the research skills that had served me well as a journalist and acquainted myself with the fundamentals of various therapeutic modalities. On learning that Freud was associated with psychoanalysis and psychodynamic training, I immediately rejected the idea of training in this modality, such was the impact and legacy of his demonisation during my psychology modules at university. As I read more, however, the idea of the unconscious and the influence of its processes continued to call to me for reasons I do not think I even comprehended at the time. Eventually, I set my prejudices aside and decided that psychodynamic training was the one for me. I became consciously aware of this interest especially in relation to my work over the last seven or eight years. (I have been a practicing counsellor now for 14 years.)

Whilst working in a university setting, I was seeing increasing numbers of young people presenting with mood disorders. Many still in or barely out of their teens had long-term enduring diagnoses of depression and anxiety. (There is plenty of documented evidence that the two usually co-exist, one taking precedent in many cases.) I also started to notice during the assessment that there was often a history of some form of transgenerational trauma within the family. After a while, I started to be curious about whether there may be a link between the events and experiences clients mentioned when outlining their family history and their own current mental and emotional states.

I was hearing tales not only of various trauma within the family that dated back generations but also of ways in which they appeared to be manifesting in current generations. For instance, a client's grandfather may have been a war survivor whose mother experienced him as distant, unavailable and perhaps unpredictable emotionally, and so the client's mother may now be someone who experiences severe anxiety and maybe depression as well. The client in turn has a diagnosis of anxiety and depression. These young clients also often reported issues with regulating emotion, usually relaying that they were quite simply at a loss as to how to manage certain feelings and would often indicate that they would really rather not have them at all, even implying that they were hoping therapy would provide a way to eradicate such feelings. After coming across this repeatedly, I could not help wondering about threads of unprocessed, unspoken trauma being communicated between the generations.

My own experience of transgenerational trauma had taught me that we share what our parents and grandparents have experienced whether they tell us or not. What we observe in them informs our internal processes and ways of being. This "simmering awareness" as described by Eva Hoffman, a second-generation war survivor ... explains that we affect each other in ways both immediate and invisible ... mental states are communicated ... not only through rational messages but along unconscious channels (Ikeda, 2014: 47).

Based on the experience and knowledge I had acquired both through my practice to that point and holding in mind ideas around unconscious processes including unconscious communication (as described by Freud and Klein), as well as ideas around how unprocessed emotions may manifest, I began to enquire and explore with clients what messages or communications they felt they may have received regarding emotions. By this I mean, on a fundamental level, what communication (both conscious and unconscious) has been internalised around feelings especially those deemed to be more challenging such as sadness, fear, and anger? What have clients noticed those around them doing with their feelings and how in turn do they think this has impacted them (the client)?

With clients who recount tales of multiple trauma in relation to their parents and grandparents and/or report struggling with managing emotions I often enquire about the messages they received by saying something along the lines of:

> The way we learn about emotions is similar to how we learn to talk. Without being aware of it, we observe, collect information from those around us and gradually we start to speak. What do you think you may have observed from those around you about what to do with feelings? What have you noticed they do with theirs and how does that affect what you do with yours?

At this point in the conversation, clients often pause as this may not be something they have reflected on before. When they stop to think about it, they begin to make the links for themselves. It is not uncommon for clients to say things like:

> Well, my dad doesn't do anything with his feelings, he just doesn't talk about things, he bottles them up whereas my mum is more open although she can be anxious. Now I think about it, I'm more like my dad.

To facilitate further exploration, I may ask follow-up questions such as "I wonder what you mean by bottling up" and/or "what impact, if any, do you think this has on how you see feelings?" This can often lead to an interesting conversation about their perceptions around feelings including how or whether to express them and why they think those perceptions exist.

During these conversations I am frequently left wondering about the notion of "simmering awareness" and what information has been shared (processed and unprocessed, spoken and unspoken) between the generations currently stopping with the client. I am reminded that being a second or even third-generation trauma survivor is almost like being part of a confusing game of Chinese whispers, quite often with no whispers. Information is received in a kind of garbled form; feelings are generated that often affect one's way of being and one is left to process and navigate this second-hand information for the sake of one's own wellbeing whilst attending sensitively to the needs of the originator (if they are still living that is). It's all something of a quagmire.

In my case, my mother's openness and willingness to discuss her experiences (partly because she needed to so that she could process them) means that I have a lot of the information I need to help me understand and situate my various responses and emotions. Despite this, however it can still be challenging at times distinguishing and locating what belongs to me and what is legacy driven and maybe that is the point. In many ways it is all interconnected and for it to be any other way would be a loss of its own.

Writing this, I am reminded of my mother's reaction when I first told her about Chimamanda Ngozi Adichie's famous breakout novel *Half of a Yellow Sun*. I told her this novel was based around the Biafran War and that I was keen to read it, primarily from my perspective for information and out of curiosity about something that was part of my history. My usually good-natured mother reacted with such vehement objection saying "What does she know about it? Was she there?" that I immediately dropped the subject and never brought it up again nor have I read the book to this day.

There are so many things to unpick here. Chimamanda being an Igbo person is presumably, like me, a second-generation Biafran survivor and this probably drove her in some way to write this book. That aside however, I think that single event more than any other conversation I ever had with my mother about the Biafran war conveyed to me the depth of the pain and trauma she had experienced. This usually good-natured encouraging woman, enthusiastic about literature and Igbo culture but also supportive of me and my pursuits and interests, shut that conversation down in a way that I knew it could not be revisited. This was not how I usually experienced my mother. The deep-seated wound I sensed in that encounter has always stayed with me.

I am also reminded of Ikeda's suggestion (1994) that written texts do not sufficiently convey the impact of war on survivors and that narratives can offer a somewhat skewed perspective of events depending on the writer. I guess in documenting an event such as the Biafran War, there are bound to be missing and competing narratives and looking back, I think my mother found it galling that someone else, especially someone who had not experienced it first hand, was essentially documenting her story. My unwitting lack of sensitivity in inviting her to partake in this narrative reminds me of when well-meaning people in my life (often Caucasian) enthusiastically tell me about a book they've read or (more often) a film or documentary they have seen about some form of racial injustice especially in the wake of George Floyd's death. They extol its virtues and recommend I watch it. If only I had a pound for each time, I had to explain that it may not necessarily be something I want to do because for me it is not just a form of education, entertainment, or information but a possible source of re-traumatisation.

Being a Black woman living in the West and being of Nigerian Igbo descent means for me the layers of transgenerational trauma run deep. The legacies of colonialism, imperialism, and racial injustice are also part of my history and I navigate these in various ways every day. These well-meaning forms of media, although helpful to an extent in documenting stories and events, can also foster the idea that we are homogenous without unique identities and individual stories to tell. The subject of identity is one that is often prevalent in my work with young people from an ethnic minority and especially Black identifying background.

According to the ideas of social constructionism the ways in which the social group to which we belong is regarded by wider society can impact not just our sense of self but our experiences of the world (Gergen, 1999). So what happens when the messages we receive from our families and wider society about who we are and who we should be are at odds with who we actually are? What happens when one is bound by one's desires but feels a (conscious or unconscious) sense of being pulled towards maintaining the narrative within which they have been constructed? This could be linked to what Freud refers to as an intrapsychic conflict, where competing and opposing factors in one's inner world potentially create distress and confusion.

A very simple example of this can be a young ethnic minority client being afraid to introduce their parents to their Caucasian partner. Exploration of this can reveal anxiety around being seen as a "coconut" (white on the inside, brown on the outside) by their family and community but also of their conscious or unconscious sense of betrayal of their ethnic group especially given the history of colonialism and imperialism. Are they now identifying with the oppressor? Then there are the societal optics and the way in which, for example, Black women are socially constructed as either less than desirable than their other counterparts or fetishised objects with not much intellectual capacity. This may well make the young person question their otherwise seemingly attentive, kind, and loving partner's real motives for being with her. There is so much here to unpack about the self: the self in relation to societal expectation, the self as a person who bears their own desires, and the self as a young person in love with someone from a culture that represents a legacy of pain for previous generations of one's ancestors and the self as part of a collective. Identity being rooted in one's position within the collective is one that is very common in non-Western societies and a concept that can sometimes be pathologised in therapy when approached from a purely Euro-Centric perspective.

Of course, all our identities are to some extent rooted within our history, both familial and societal. However, in many non-Western cultures one's position in the family's system and how that position is perceived plays a large part in constructing individual identity. In situations where there is a legacy of trauma, there is a sense (in my experience) of the descending generations being the vessel for various processes including attempts at articulation, enactment, reparation, and a conduit between the past and future generations. Holding that position whether willingly or unwillingly, consciously or unconsciously, is woven into the fabric of one's identity. Learning to decipher what processes may be theirs, what may be inherited, and how to navigate and engage with feelings can often make a real difference to our clients' inner world and overall state of mind. Equally acknowledging that the inherited and individual are irrevocably intertwined and not everything can be made sense of can sometimes be the key to reconciling intrapsychic conflicts.

When beginning with clients I often explain the way I work partly using an analogy borrowed from my first supervisor which I have expanded on over the years. I tell them that I see the processes of their inner world as something of a jigsaw puzzle. As the expert on their own life, they possess the pieces, and it is my role to sit or walk alongside them as they put the puzzle together. We may not locate all the pieces or indeed be able to place their locations (stressing that this is okay and it can be torturous and distracting trying) but we can get enough of an image to understand why they are where they are now and what they might need to do to make a shift.

In describing this I am acknowledging not only the client's ability to locate and process their experiences but also that some things are either so out of awareness or difficult to locate that pursuing them may not only be a distraction but exacerbate distress. What we know or discover can be incredibly powerful as it can inform our next steps. Equally, accepting with compassion for ourselves and others that there are things which impact us which may always remain unconscious but also intrinsically a part of us can help us to let go of the search to make the unknown known and start building with what we do have. As I have seen with clients, when this position is reached, a shift can occur which usually brings with it some sense of liberation, acceptance, and agency.

I would like to clarify that I am by no means stating that this is the case for everyone who experiences issues with their mood and mental health, their identity, or indeed has had experience of transgenerational trauma as every individual is as unique as they are complex. In my experience, however, these ideas do seem to resonate and support a large proportion of clients when exploring and attempting to make sense of their inner world. I also feel that there does not necessarily have to have been a history of significant trauma for these ideas to be relevant although one could argue that any life lived over a certain span will encounter some trauma. The people in our lives, especially those who play some role in shaping and nurturing our sense of self, invariably influence the way we see and feel about the world and ourselves in ways that we do not always even fully recognise or comprehend. Developing an understanding of how this can manifest and having some tools to navigate this is one of the ways in which we equip ourselves for living.

Another way in which my experience of transgenerational trauma impacts my work is in my thinking with clients around family dynamics and their relationships, particularly with parents. Over the years, I have encountered many clients whose levels of distress and sense of self have been significantly impacted by what they view to be unfeeling parents who appear to make no attempt at emotional connection, leaving the client feeling wounded and distant from their parent(s). Often through exploration, they start to join up the dots for themselves and see the transgenerational or environmental and relational links that may be impacting on their interactions with their parents.

An example of this could be whilst working with a client who over the course of relaying their experiences of their distant mother who they feel has never shown any real interest in them other than the perfunctory; I may ask how the mother interacts with her parents and perhaps others in their life. At this point there is often a pause for thought and the client might say something like "Well, my grandad was never really around and I think my grandma suffered from depression her whole life so my mum never really had much of a relationship with them". I may say something such as, "it sounds like she may have been lonely and had to rely on herself a fair bit" to which the client may reply "I guess so". I then ask, "how do you think this may have affected how she is with people?" To which the client may say "Well, I guess she holds back".

Over the course of this exchange, the client is able to explore and gain insight into how their mother's history may be influencing her interactions with others, and upon further reflection they may realise that there are other ways in which she demonstrates love and affection which they had never previously noticed or acknowledged. In gaining some understanding of the legacy of their parent's history (and arguably) trauma, the client in this example has an opportunity to make sense of the impact this has had on their parent's interactions with them and in doing so develops a new sense of understanding and empathy for their parent. This new-found empathy could in turn lead to a more open and forgiving way of being on the part of the client which could over time lead them closer to that more affectionate and connected relationship they had been seeking.

As I end this, I am reminded of two sayings: Winnicott's declaration that "there is no such thing as a baby, only a nursing couple" and the famous proverb "it takes a village to raise a child". What both these observations have in common is their indication that each generation requires the nurturing support and knowledge of the previous generation in order to develop and, hopefully, thrive. In performing this function however, all aspects of knowledge and history belonging to the previous generation are passed down. In other words, the good is integrated with the bad, the painful with the joyous. To split these would be what Klein refers to as the paranoid schizoid position resulting in relationships which lack authenticity and that deny aspects of one's identity.

The trick, however, is to find one's way of navigating all that history and its legacy in a way that acknowledges its significance and value but equally allows the present to take a shape of its own in a way that feels authentic to the individual. After all, if it was not for the Biafran War and the way in which it changed the course of my parents' lives (especially my mother's) I would likely be living an entirely different life. Amidst the pain, I am aware of the gifts it has given me. Having an inherent understanding of the wounding but also the courage, compassion, and strength that can accompany the human condition have equipped me for many aspects of my life and work. Over time, I have learned to be with the past in a way that allows it and me to live together in the present.

References

Freud, S (1923) *The Ego and the Id*. In the Standard Edition of the Complete Psychological Works of Sigmund Freud (vol. 19) (ed Strachey, J): 13–27. London. Hogarth Press.

Gergen, K (1999) *An Invitation to Social Construction*. London. Sage Publishing.

Hoffman, E (2004) *After Such Knowledge: Memory, History and the Legacy of the Holocaust*. New York. Public Affairs cited in: Ikeda, K (2014) *Okinawan War Memory: Transgenerational Trauma and the War Fiction of Medoruma Shun*. New York. Routledge.

Ikeda, K (2014) *Okinawan War Memory: Transgenerational Trauma and the War Fiction of Medoruma Shun*. New York. Routledge.

Jung, CG (1968) *The Archetypes and the Collective Unconscious*. (2nd Edition). London. Routledge.

Klein, M (1997) *Envy and Gratitude and Other Works 1946–1963*. London. Vintage.

Chapter 7

Sibling death

Mourning in childhood and beyond

Josephine Evans

The death of a young person is always a tragic event which resonates deeply and profoundly with domino effects for years to come, if not for lifetimes. This is the central theme of this chapter which focuses on the enduring impact of grief on my family following the loss of my brother, the youngest child, with particular reference to how it affected me at the time and what we can learn from this traumatic family event about the adolescent experience of sibling death more generally. This event was shaped in the context of our white, middle-class family in the 1970s when the response to a death, and the provision of support, was entirely different from today. I will reflect on how the death of a child in a family 50 years ago was experienced, both internally and externally, but in my case remained undigested for decades. This will be linked with contemporary examples from my therapeutic work in schools with bereaved siblings.

Looking through a societal and historical lens, I will go further back in time to explore the impact of earlier sibling bereavements experienced by my grandparents. Their stories were woven into the fabric of my family history, albeit often with threads almost too fine to detect. I will reflect upon how earlier unarticulated sibling losses such as that of my grandmother can filter through the generations even if this is unspoken and only 'felt' within the shadows.

My own experience

These days I can say to people, when asked, that I'm the middle child of three and that when I was 11 my younger brother died aged eight of a malignant brain tumour. For years I grappled with the uncomfortable question – 'to tell or not to tell?' – about this momentous experience. Either way I would be faced with a painful dilemma. Keeping silent meant being guilty of betrayal in failing to acknowledge my brother's existence while speaking up risked uninvited responses, ranging from shock and surprise or intense curiosity through to rapid and awkward conversational backpedalling.

The subsequent ripple effect of my brother's short illness and death (spanning four months before Christmas in 1978), coinciding with my transition to secondary school, has shaped my developing self, influencing who and what I

DOI: 10.4324/9781003270447-8

have become in adult life. There was no such thing as counselling in schools in the 1970s, and with all the 'what ifs' and 'if onlys' I can only imagine how different my journey might have been had there been a thinking space provided at the time to try and make sense of this traumatic event. A sibling is 'ingrained in us' and 'intertwined in our shared DNA', even though bereaved siblings have been referred to as the 'forgotten mourners' (Hayes, 2018). My brother's death was life-changing and pivotal, but the usual and familiar family routines continued undisturbed. However, I was acutely aware of a creeping sense of unease that the status quo could never again be trusted and relied upon; all of life's certainties that had previously been taken for granted were open to question. As Balk describes, the crisis shook, if not shattered, assumptions about the predictability of the world. (Balk, 2014, 33).

I have referred elsewhere to the nuances in feelings relating to sibling death (Evans, 2015, 98) where a sibling alliance, known to be 'fragile and reversible' (Lowy, 2017a, 86) can feel as if permanently severed. For the surviving sibling, the opportunity for this potentially life-long relationship to 'transform itself throughout childhood, adolescence, and adult life' is denied (ibid., 2017b, 84). When my brother died, the tangible, ongoing, everyday connection with him was abruptly cut off in situ, as if interrupting one of our many disagreements. The normal process of grief seemed to exist in a suspended, never-ending time-void. As an 11-year-old, I did not have the emotional or cognitive capacities to understand, grieve, and find a place for this experience (Miles, 2010, 4). Instead, I had a sense that grief was reserved for adults; it remained out of sight and earshot but occasionally popped up unnervingly like a Jack-in-the-box. My own loss became an unacknowledged fog tucked away in a frozen rupture of space and time (Coles, 2011, 34), further complicated by residual feelings of envy towards my dead brother, with whom my conflicts remained 'alive and kicking' in the narrative of my internal world. My guilty triumph over his death was also marred by a double bind of resentment towards what I perceived to be his now eternally elevated status as the 'golden boy'. Survivor's guilt can manifest in many ways. In my case, an internal record kept spinning, giving me the message that in order to justify this loss, my life would have to be doubly worthwhile and have intrinsic value; that there was no time to waste because life as I now knew it was fleeting. These floating thoughts influenced my successive life choices, but even so, it felt a betrayal to claim and celebrate my successes in my first profession as an actor/musician. In my distorted mind's eye, my brother was the natural entertainer who would have excelled in this career; I was only able to take up this role as his death left a vacancy.

I know from my research into adolescent bereavement that a 'positive outcome for … survivors of sibling death … occurs when, in an attempt to adapt to the loss and its symbolic reparation, they structure their careers accordingly' (Lowry, 2017a, 89 referencing Oltjenbruns, 1991). Having finally faced the shadow of grief which had accompanied me, unacknowledged for decades, I became part of the 'wounded healer' community of therapists for which the above quote applies (Jung, 1993). My first profession was a less conscious choice, but I would suggest no less relevant in this sense. In retrospect I can see how I was drawn to the world of entertainment to compensate for our family loss, as a way of outwardly trying to enliven and distract us from the undercurrent of pain. Performing 'in character' provided a space for me to explore and discharge intense feelings whilst being 'one step removed' behind the theatrical mask. I relished the artistic precision and stamina required to create certainty within the known parameters of a show, in contrast to my belief that 'real life' was fickle and unpredictable. I took up a role of filling the space created in a show symbolically to fill the internal void left in the wake of my brother's death.

The sense of quiet dread which accompanied my development into adulthood was impossible to keep carefully under wraps when I became a parent during my thirties. This was the trigger which meant that feelings deeply buried could no longer be denied, and I sought therapy for the first time. I was shocked to discover irrational but seemingly unstoppable thoughts, willing my daughters to live beyond their eighth birthdays, echoing the view that 'death anxiety is another reported long-term outcome of sibling loss ... there is also a fear of recurrence of the loss' (Miles, 2010, 13). In this way, 'a dead sibling can take possession of a family', by casting a trajectory of grief over subsequent generations (Coles, 2011, 41). This is a theme I return to when I look at my grandparents' experiences of sibling loss (below) and how this remained an unspoken but felt presence in the years to follow.

Within and without – working with a young person going through a recent sibling bereavement

Personal therapy offered me the opportunity to explore in depth the build-up of feelings which had resided within, unabsorbed, both in mind and body. This process enabled me to contemplate moving from a 'stuck' place to a greater understanding of the felt experience of grief in childhood and adolescence. My interest in the subject gradually expanded beyond my own history, leading in time to my decision to train in this field. However, there have been times during my role as an adolescent counsellor and psychotherapist, when I have worked with bereaved students whose experiences have appeared (at least on the face of it) closely akin to my own. In these instances, certain details emerging from the referral and subsequent sessions can accentuate aspects of my past which require further consideration in relation to the work.

This was particularly so when working with a Year 7 student named Sade, who was referred to me for counselling as her younger brother was terminally ill. Her situation uncannily reflected mine, including my age at the time of my brother's illness and subsequent death, although her family configuration, cultural heritage, and ancestry were entirely different from my own. However, I was very much aware in my own pre-transference to our face-to-face work that I was preoccupied with our seemingly analogous experiences. This necessitated careful reflection in supervision, which involved re-visiting the material from my own past to sift through some of the complexities surrounding my brother's death. A particularly uncomfortable feeling requiring attention was that of my own envy towards Sade. I found myself musing over the differences in how bereavement was responded to within schools then and now.

Nonetheless, in anticipation of our first session, I was still wrangling with my own historical context, including some ambivalence about whether I could keep my story in the background, maintaining my 'analytic discretion' while also making space for my own subjectivities (Kuchuck, 2014). Could I attend to Sade's direct experience with an 'evenly hovering attention' (Freud, 1909)? Or would I be in danger of overidentifying with her narrative and consequently be less attuned to the differences? I suspect that I'm not the only therapist to wrestle with questions of this ilk. Looking back at my experience in the light of Sade's highlighted the scant support I received at that time. I recall being summoned to the Headteacher's office, alongside another student who was being praised for his excellent artwork. The Headteacher asked me drily, in front of the other pupil, 'how are things at home?' I automatically replied that everything was 'fine' when life felt anything but. My brother's illness and imminent death were not mentioned again in school. This was not unusual for the time. I am simply a statistic of my generation: 'No-one had ever asked [us] what it was like to be the sibling of someone who had died' (Miles, 3, 2010).

Sade's experience would be wholly dissimilar from mine in this respect. Counselling was offered by the school before her sibling died, which provided the opportunity for pre-bereavement work with her. It was possible to begin establishing a therapeutic relationship and to prepare her for ongoing support that could unfold at her own pace. This required sensitively gauging Sade's readiness to engage with any thinking in the immediate aftermath of her loss, recognising that the disorientating and raw knowledge of a recent death will move in and out of focus and up and down the emotional register. This was originally described by Freud as a gradual 'bit by bit' painful and slow struggle to accept the death (Malawista, 2017, 38).

A careful balance had to be struck between keeping a space open for reflection, while at the same time respecting Sade's need for her defences. The timing and frequency of sessions offered were negotiated with Sade's preferences in mind. Managing emotional intensity was important as our work was taking place in school and Sade needed to be ready to return to class at the end of each session. I also had to consider whether the more complicated process of thinking about and trying to make sense of a death was an appropriate intervention to offer while Sade was still in the midst of the experience. Bereaved young people need day-to-day school routines which provide a reassuring sense that 'normal life' is still possible. The ordinary everydayness of school serves as a temporary distraction from an inescapable home environment, one which, in Sade's case, was dominated first by the anticipation of her brother's death and then its aftermath. Just as significantly, school offered her respite from witnessing her parents' sometimes very raw grief.

Following her brother's death, the flurry of sympathetic well-wishers and preparations for the funeral left very little space for reflection. At the same time, there was almost too much potential for emotional investment by others. As this tragic event unfolded, Sade dreaded being faced each day with concerned staff and students asking how she was, feeling 'put on the spot' in each instance, and at risk of being 'found out', where becoming overwhelmed threatened exposure and further unwanted curiosity. Thinking about the death of her sibling at this stage felt 'too much' for Sade. The time when counselling seemed most helpful came later when the painful reality of her brother's absence was keenly and unavoidably felt. Our sessions offered Sade a place to bring her sense of rage and confusion, to a greater or lesser degree, depending on whether these feelings were able to be borne by her. For my part, I needed to stay in touch with the reality of Sade's loss yet approach our sessions with a degree of flexibility so that I could better attune to Sade's needs and let her set the pace.

Parental loss from a young person's perspective

The journey of grief can cause us to flip backwards and forwards in time, a process that remains unendingly in a state of flux. Recovery of a previous self is not possible; however hard we try to regain what was, there will always be a sense of unfinished business, even if this runs alongside some kind of acceptance. Writing this has caused me to revisit the details of how my immediate family members experienced my brother's death. It was 30 years before we sat down and talked together about our individual and collective responses. Even though this meeting was safely couched in the guise of 'research' as part of my therapy training, we were able to discuss our own (surprisingly differing) timelines and outlooks, illustrating how the 'facts' of an event can be enduringly wrapped up in our own frame of reference (Rogers, 1980, 140).

An overriding sense of desolation mingled with shame can set off 'a chain reaction of connected lives damaged' by 'the jagged, unpredictable nature of grief' (Haig, 10th November 2007). For most parents, losing a child causes 'a rupture that cannot be repaired' (Smolen, 2017, 125). It is every parent's worst living nightmare, so much so that the wider community can be at a loss as to how to deal with such a tragedy, even superstitiously fearing 'contamination' and a kind of 'collective shame' that this has happened within their circle. This was certainly a factor in our experience in the 1970s though perhaps to a lesser degree in the present day where displays of grief have become more accessible (for example, the collective nationwide grief-stricken response to the death of Diana, Princess of Wales). As an 11-year-old, I was aware that some acquaintances seemed eager to 'fix' things, with the proverbial 'cup of tea' being offered as something that could help. Some seemed to struggle with what might be the most appropriate thing to say, when perhaps 'there but for the grace of God' was writ large in their thoughts. I overheard comments intended to reassure such as, 'at least you have two other children', and was also aware of my brother's death being carefully circumvented in passing conversations. Some even crossed to the other side of the street to avoid direct contact with us. In this way, the bereaved can feel ousted and left with a sense of their own 'contagion', compounded by the all-pervading unvoiced dynamic of a subject which remains off-limits.

One may also imagine shared familial loss as a 'uniting process' (Haig, 6th November 2007), but in fact the opposite can also occur, where 'it polarises and separates the bereaved' (ibid., 2007). Our family had tried to survive the emotional rollercoaster of our shared tragedy by retreating into protective bubbles of solitude. This had taken us via the short-lived hope of some kind of recovery for my brother, following the shock of his collapse, to the crushing and re-traumatising realisation in the face of his subsequent rapid deterioration, that his condition was terminal.

At the time, much as our parents tried to protect my older brother and me from the intensity of their grief, this remained viscerally present in the household. I sensed that my mother took her grief elsewhere, sometimes heading out in the car on her own. In our family conversation that I facilitated three decades later, she acknowledged that this was indeed the case as she thought that her overwhelming feelings would frighten us: 'I wasn't just dabbing my eyes, dear, I was shrieking in utter agony'. She'd become pre-occupied with her work and keeping herself busy with home-based projects such as having a new kitchen installed, telling me all those years later that 'I had a choice: to give up or to keep going'. She also tried to find some explanation for the seemingly random event of my brother's death as there had only ever been one other recorded case of a child under ten with a brain haemorrhage precipitating a 'high-grade glioma' (a tumour that originates in the glial cells of the brain). In her desperate search for an answer, she frequently chastised herself for once travelling near to the Sellafield Nuclear Plant during her pregnancy.

In that same conversation, my father described a physical process of grief which only started to abate after two years, where his pain caused him to curl into a foetal position, as if 'bent double' by the intensity of feeling. Again, I was aware of this being part of my parents' experience of mourning which they attempted to hide from us children, but nonetheless, my brother and I witnessed moments of unabridged grief which were at times unavoidable. Both parents talked about the physical need to release feelings of anguish. They were able to keep this at bay during everyday interactions but said that it always returned, arriving with what they described as an automatic grip like a big black cloud which pressed down on them although they knew at the end, they could come back up out of it. This was something they both saw as cathartic and necessary.

My parents' 'conscious decision to survive' a loss which was so illogical in every way, and described by my father as a 'genetic outrage, forging against the laws of nature', spurred their grief into action (Talbot, 2002). Even though in one sense any potential for the future had been in my father's words 'ripped out', there was a semblance of an idea that to proactively fight back in the face of grief would help them to maintain some sense of meaning. Amongst other things they organised a committee to create a Memorial Fund in my brother's name to raise money for Cancer Research, making sponsored walks, jumble sales, and concerts a dominant part of our weekends. They also instigated a project for a new commemorative stained-glass window to be installed in the local church. It was as if their grief knew no bounds as they pushed through bureaucratic ecclesiastical hoops to achieve this. But one of the legacies and compromises of 'keeping going' was to perpetuate an avoidance of looking back, as well as a sidestep around processing, understanding, and ultimately accepting this unbearable reality.

An attempt to leave grief behind

From my clinical practice over the years I have also been made aware of the parental impetus to sustain some sense of purpose in life, following the death of their child. This can take various forms (as with my own parents) including a decision to move home. For some families, the stimulus of relocating can serve to distract from the intolerable, constant reminder of their dead child's absence. This has been the case with some of the young people I have worked with. They were rarely consulted about moving house, and in each instance, they shared with me ambivalent feelings of relief and deep regret that their shared sibling history was being left behind at this point of no return.

A Year 9 boy, Toby, experienced the death of his older brother (aged 16 and preparing for his impending GCSE examinations) who had died during the night with no warning of any previous health issues. The death was subsequently and inconclusively attributed to Sudden Arrhythmic Death Syndrome. It was a deeply traumatic event for Toby, compounded by the painful awareness that his older brother had died in his sleep on the bunk bed beneath him. During the ensuing panic when paramedics were unable to revive his brother, Toby was distressingly in touch with the horror of his own and his parents' helplessness.

The school was keen to offer him 'rapid response' support and in this instance, I was aware of Toby's need not only to recount the vivid details he'd witnessed, but also initially to share and repeat his story, as if to confirm every time the dreadful reality of what had happened. It felt as if this enabled him to place himself within his own process and experience, although the inexplicable mystery surrounding the death of his perfectly healthy teenage brother felt unacceptable and beyond belief. There was now a void stretching out before him which had been filled with the anticipation of their shared future together. This empty space would now have to be filled by Toby who found himself in the position of eldest child and would be the first, and not the second, to take GCSEs and leave home to go to university.

As our sessions continued, I heard of his parents' plan to move home. It quickly became evident that this decision was taken to leave behind the daily visual cues of their trauma. It appeared that Toby and his other younger siblings were not consulted in this push to turn away from what was unbearable for the parents. This felt disorientating for him, as if the narrative of their formative years in this house including birthday celebrations, games of hide and seek, racing down the corridor and so on, were being wiped out against the backdrop of their loss. It felt to him too drastic a move to leave all this behind, and he insisted upon taking the bunk beds to the family's new home. Even though his brother's death meant that Toby now had his own bedroom, the physical presence of the bunkbeds seemed to enable him to retain a felt connection with his brother. Remaining on the top bunk with the now empty bed below allowed Toby to imagine for a few moments on waking that everything was as 'normal', that his brother was still asleep in the bunk beneath. The bottom bunk also served to help him bear manageable waves of grief by sitting there from time to time, 'but not for too long'.

The death of a sibling jolts our perception of our self in the world bringing in its wake a new proximity to our own mortality. There can be a sense of being disenfranchised and cast adrift in infinity with an interruption of our previously secure space and time construct. This eclipses a seemingly blissful ignorance of the time before, when the idea of our own death may not have been in conscious awareness. As expressed by the actor, comedian, and cartoonist Jessie Cave following her brother's death: 'You're not living the same life anymore … it's so hard to accept … I'm surprised by how brutal it is, that separation of before and after' (2021).

Historical sibling bereavements

Traumatic loss going back generations can span time, residing glancingly in the shadows of the present, almost within reach but not quite. There were several sibling deaths relating to my grandparents' younger years which were mentioned occasionally during my upbringing, but it is only more recently that new details have come to light via newspaper articles and letters. Two of these sibling deaths were the result of tragic accidents; entirely unprepared for and seemingly random events which became 'the kind that are unseen … they don't have … substance, but they have impact … They represent the voices of the past' (Dr. Anat, 2012).

Great aunt Lucy

I recently found a family album belonging to my maternal grandmother which shows two photographs side by side. The location is identical, although the dates show they were each taken a year apart. In both pictures, my grandmother smiles at the camera, kneeling beside a pond of waterlilies. In the first picture, her younger sister is at her side, however she is absent in the second. Had I not subsequently discovered details of the traumatic loss which occurred in the time between these photographs, there would be nothing here to suggest that a tragedy took place in the interval between these sun-drenched scenes.

In the ether of distant family conversations, I remember hearing that my grandmother's sister Lucy had been killed in a bicycling accident. Two generations later and never having known her in person, it felt as if her presence was nurtured in my grandmother's re-telling of their close filial bond. Nearly a century later after my great aunt's death, I find myself researching the details, prompted by writing this chapter. A local newspaper described 'a poignant tragedy' of a 'husband's three days bedside vigil' of a 'twenty-five-year-old girl ... three months married ... where hosts of friends [were] plunged into sorrow at her death' (Fleetwood Chronicle, 28th December 1928). It appeared that Lucy had fallen off her bicycle and landed under a milk float, suffering a fatal head injury. She died three days later, on Christmas Day, following an unsuccessful operation to 'remove a small piece of bone and a clot of blood ... from her skull' (ibid., 1928).

I can only wonder how Lucy's death affected subsequent Christmases for my grandmother. With each passing year following my brother's death I have grown to appreciate how important it is to acknowledge anniversaries. As a rite of passage, an annual visit to his graveside either on the day he died or on his birthday has for the most part continued over the years to the present day. This has become a familiar, contemplative, and unforeseeably containing place to return to, sometimes with existing or subsequent family members, but mostly now by myself.

This ritual does also frequently come up in my work when bereaved young people talk about their plans for the pending anniversary of a death, often with feelings of reluctance, awkwardness, and a sense of obligation. If a family is struggling to articulate and communicate their shared loss with each other, the graveside vigil can lull them into an uncomfortable silence or a surface preoccupation with arranging the flowers, or pulling up the weeds, all to 'smooth over the rough edges'. Christmases felt like something to be endured in the years following my brother's death, and for my grandmother, so deeply affected by the loss of her grandson almost exactly 50 years after that of her sister, this time must have triggered memories and feelings of her previous loss, albeit unknown to me.

Great uncle Thomas

I have also had cause lately to sift through some previously unseen diaries belonging to my parents and grandmother. The one that they all kept and documented was for 1978, the year of my brother's death. There is even a pocket diary belonging to my brother for that year, with his handwriting marking the dates of our pending summer holiday that was cancelled owing to his illness. Concrete evidence of a life can be stashed away in a cupboard for decades, remaining as fragments of an existence which otherwise can only reside in the mind as a collection of memories, and musings of what could have been. Ann G. Smolen writes about this experience, saying that,

> No matter the age of the child or whether the child dies suddenly or after a prolonged terminal illness the end result is the same: Those who are left are devastated. When a very young child dies, there is often a desire and yearning to imagine what type of older child and adult he would have become.
>
> (Smolen, 2017, 126)

A pocket notebook bearing my 16-year-old great uncle Thomas' name and handwriting was one of the only pieces of tangible proof available to identify his body, found face-down in the sea off the coast of Bangor. He was wearing 'blue corded serge', which matched the 'missing passengers' description released some weeks beforehand (Larne Times and Weekly Telegraph, 28th July 1900). Thomas had been visiting his grandparents in Glenarm (County Antrim) and was travelling back on the 'Dromedary' steamer via Belfast Lough to re-join his family in Glasgow. He had boarded at Belfast Docks, but with 'awful suddenness ... an impenetrable fog ... dropped ... like a screen' (Northern Whig, Monday 23rd July 1900), and caused the vessel to collide at full speed with the 'Alligator' steamer travelling in the opposite direction. Thomas's body was one of the last to be found. When the cause of the accident was 'thrashed out in court' (Belfast Evening Telegraph, 10th August 1900) at the inquest, it was surmised that he must have drowned, having been 'thrown overboard' (ibid., 1900) on impact.

The news reaching Glasgow was received 'with feelings of profound consternation and alarm' and 'anxious dread' (The Northern Whig, Monday, 23rd July 1900). Apparently, there were frantic scrambles at the dock and the hospitals where families desperately tried to find out about survivors. I wondered whether my ancestors were part of these scenes. It is hard to imagine how they reacted when the realisation that Thomas was missing penetrated through the shock and disbelief. Looking at the dates I am aware that his mother had either just had a baby or was due to give birth at that time. My paternal grandfather was eight, one of four other brothers who later survived WW1. Thomas's life had been cut short en route to his joyfully anticipated return, alluded to in the tantalising detail that 'a large bouquet of peculiar form which the deceased had been carrying had been found' (Belfast Evening Telegraph, 10th August 1900). Perhaps this was meant as a gift for his mother or even to celebrate the arrival of another brother. The loss was felt on an immediate and community level, where 'to remember the desolated homes and broken hearts caused by this disaster, and to think of the pain and anguish many a humble person had suffered, and of the blighted and ruined lives caused by it' (Belfast Evening Telegraph, 8th August 1900), brings this intense experience of shared grief into sharp present-day focus.

It is not possible to find out how the surviving siblings experienced the shock of their brother Thomas' death, and how the news 'landed' within their family. However, I am aware that until around 50 years ago it was generally believed that children did not have the capacity to understand the concept of death, let alone the ability to grieve. It was considered best to leave them 'completely in the dark' (Miles, 2010, 9). I am left wondering how the devastating impact of Thomas' death could have been hidden from his siblings, living as they did in a cramped tenement flat, if this was the case. I cannot imagine that the trajectory of grief, unbound by human constraints of time, place and history was not felt in this instance of sibling loss. Be it 1900, 1928, 1978, or the present day, the lateral, enduring life span of a continued sibling bond does not end with their death. An abiding 'wish to stay connected with our deceased sibling may grow with the years rather than decrease' (Miles, 2010, 18). This is certainly true for me, as with other bereaved siblings with whom I have come into contact. I can only assume this to be true of my paternal grandfather, and maternal grandmother as well.

I feel a greater sense of relatedness to my great uncle and aunt since these facts have emerged, despite knowing very little about my grandmother's sister, and having never met my grandfather, who died before I was born. My father had only mentioned in passing that his uncle had drowned, an event he placed firmly in the past even though for me it reverberates so strongly as I write.

Conclusion

In this chapter, I have been exploring separation and loss from the perspective of sibling bereavement, connecting histories of the past and present with reference to my work as a school-based therapist. The loss of a sibling has been described as '… a grievous one and mobilises deep and painful mourning' (Lowry, 2017b, 86). This fact has historically been overlooked until more recently. The young person going through this experience may be denied the opportunity to mourn their life-changing loss if developmentally appropriate support is not made available to them. In addition, their particular family configuration will need consideration so their loss can find a place in the context of their own personal history. If not, they risk constructing an internal narrative around the belief that their grief is inaccessible or even prohibited, and the process of mourning can become an unexplored event locked in a time warp which nonetheless lives on unvoiced in the present.

We all express loss differently, whether individually, in families or in communities; but death and ensuing grief is a universal and unavoidable fact of life however it is experienced. Grief is 'a state of being as opposed to a goal of resolution' (Miles, 2010, 32). Grief has no notion of time, hard though we try to place it in the past, and attempt to look in the opposite direction. I have highlighted my family experience of loss that occurred so many years ago, but alongside many other families who have suffered the death of a child, 'there is no real consolation, no substitution' (Smolen, 2017, 119). My brother's 'life was small his death enormous' (ibid., 135). Deaths never completely dissipate; they are embedded in family histories forever.

References

Dr.Anat. (2012). *Ghosts in the Nursery: How the Past Affects the Present.* Article from betweentherapysessions.com on Therapy Matters, referencing: Fraiberg, Selma, Adelson, Edna, Shapiro, Vivian. (1975). Ghosts in the Nursery. A Psychoanalytic Approach to the Problems of Impaired Infant-Mother Relationships. *Journal of the American Academy of Child and Adolescent Psychotherapy* 14(3), 387–421.

Balk, Davis E. (2014). *Dealing with Dying, Death and Grief during Adolescence.* London: Routledge.

Cave, Jessie. (2nd August 2021). Jessie Cave on Body Image, Bereavement and being Relentless: 'I Don't Have Any Secrets'. In: Saner, Emine (interviewer), *The G2 Interview.* London: The Guardian. https://www.theguardian.com/lifeandstyle/2021/aug/02/jessie-cave-on-body-image-bereavement-and-being-relentless-i-dont-have-any-secrets?CMP=Share_AndroidApp_Other

Coles, Prophecy. (2011). *Sibling Ghosts. The Uninvited Guest from the Unremembered Past: An Exploration of the Unconscious Transmission of Trauma Across Generations.* London: Karnac.

Evans, Josephine. (2015). 'Death of a Sibling' in Chapter 9, The Bereaved Adolescent. In: French, Lyn and Klein, Reva. (Eds.), *Therapeutic Practice in Schools Volume 2.* London: Routledge, pages 93–102.

Freud, Sigmund. (1909). *Analysis of a Phobia of a Five-Year-Old Boy.* In The Pelican Freud Library (1977), Vol 8, Case Histories 1, pages 169–306.

Haig, David. (6th November 2007). *My Boy Jack.* Interview for Front Row BBC Radio 4.

Haig, David. (10th November 2007). 'Guns and Guilt'. Preview Interview for *My Boy Jack.* timesonline.co.uk/the knowledge

Hayes, Hayley. (20th December 2018). Quoting a Bereaved Sibling during a Group Run by The Compassionate Friends in Should We Talk more about Grief? *Beyond Today.* London: Radio 4. https://www.bbc.co.uk/programmes/p06w5z3m

Jung, Carl Gustav. (1993). *The Practice of Psychotherapy. Essays on the Psychology of Transference and Other Subjects.* Collected Works of C.G. Jung. Volume 16 (works written between 1902–1961). London: Routledge.

Kuchuck, S. (2014). *Clinical Implications of the Therapist's Life Experiences: When the Personal Becomes Professional.* New York: Routledge.

Lowy, Frederick H. (2017a). Death of a Sibling (Sibling Loss in Childhood). In: Akhtar, Salman and Kanwal, Gurmeet S. (Eds.), *Bereavement: Personal Experiences and Clinical Reflections.* London: Karnac, pages 83–96.

Lowy, Frederick H. (2017b). Death of a Sibling (Nuances of Sibling Relationship). In: Akhtar, Salman and Kanwal, Gurmeet S. (Eds.), *Bereavement: Personal Experiences and Clinical Reflections.* London: Karnac.

Malawista, Kerry L. (2017). Death of a Mother. In: Akhtar, Salman and Kanwal, Gurmeet S. (Eds.), *Bereavement: Personal Experiences and Clinical Reflections.* London: Karnac, pages 33–66.

Miles, Laura Marguerite. (2010a). *Continuing Bonds: Childhood Sibling Loss and Its Perceived Long-Term Outcomes: A Project Based Upon an Independent Investigation*. Masters Thesis, Smith College, Northampton, MA. https://scholarworks.smith.edu/theses/511

Miles, Laura Marguerite. (2010b). As above. Page 9, referencing: Davies, B. (1999). *Shadows in the Sun: The Experiences of Sibling Bereavement in Childhood*. Philadelphia: Taylor & Francis.

Oltjenbruns, Kevin Ann. (1991). Positive Outcomes of Adolescent Experience with Grief. *Journal of Adolescent Research* 6, 43–53.

Rogers, Carl. (1980). *A Way of Being*. New York: Houghton Mifflin.

Smolen, Ann G. (2017). Death of a Child. In: Akhtar, Salman and Kanwal, Gurmeet S. (Eds.), *Bereavement: Personal Experiences and Clinical Reflections*. London: Karnac, pages 117–142.

Talbot, Kay. (2002). *What Forever Means After a Death of a Child: Transcending the Trauma, Living with the Loss*. London: Brunner-Routledge.

Recommended reading/bibliography

Goldman, Linda. (2022). *Life and Loss: A Guide to Help Grieving Children*. London: Routledge.

Jenkins, Clare and Merry, Judy. (2005). *Relative Grief - Parents and Children, Sisters and Brothers, Husbands, Wives and Partners, Grandparents and Grandchildren Talk About Their Experience of Death and Grieving*. London: Jessica Kingsley.

Martison, Ida M. and Campos, Rosemary Gates. (1991). Adolescent Bereavement: Long-Term Responses to a Sibling's Death from Cancer. *Journal of Adolescent Research* 6(1), 54–69.

McQuaid, Cathy. (May 2021). *Understanding Bereaved Parents and Siblings: A Handbook for Professionals, Family, and Friends*. London: Routledge.

The ABC of grief for bereaved siblings

During Cathy McQuaid's research into the experiences of bereaved parents and siblings she noticed various processes which occurred for each of the participants that she termed the ABC of Grief. This workshop introduces a model which may help understand one's own and others' processes.

Rosenfeld, Juliet. (2020). *The State of Disbelief: A Story of Death, Love and Forgetting*. London: Short Books Ltd.

Schiffman, Darin D. (2019). *Coping with the Death of a Child: An Integrated Approach to Working with Bereaved Families*. London: Routledge.

Silverman, Phyllis R. and Kelly, Madelyn. (2009). *A Parent's Guide to Raising Grieving Children: Rebuilding Your Family After the Death of a Loved One*. New York: Oxford University Press.

Chapter 8

Separation and loss in adolescence

The impact of the Iranian revolution

Farah Bajull

Writing this chapter has given me a unique opportunity to reflect on my formative years and the impact of leaving my family in Iran to study in England in 1977. At first, I felt that I had taken this journey into my past before, but as I delved deeper, I discovered that I was on a path less travelled and in internal landscapes less familiar. I stopped and started a few times along the way, unwrapping what had remained, in part, under cover for decades, pausing to process my experiences, each time confronting a different mix of emotions before I could begin writing again. What stands out most poignantly was the death of my father and the impact of this loss. I recall visiting him in the hospital for the first time after an involuntary six-year separation, and there, on his death bed, we had our long-anticipated reunion, knowing these might also be our final moments together. He was suffering from advanced lung cancer and had only had two to three months to live at best. He was so thin that I trembled with shock when I saw him, and even more so when we hugged.

My father had a traditional role as the family's protector and looked after us throughout our lives. The painful thought of a future without him seemed inconceivable. Growing up, my siblings and I idolised our father. He would occasionally summon us to sit by his side and ask how we were doing in school or talk to us about different religions and faiths, always in an unbiased way. I remember him addressing us in a gentle rather than authoritative tone.

Iran was where I spent my childhood and early adolescence. This was during the Shah's reign, prior to the 1979 Islamic revolution. I grew up in a family of five children. My brother was the oldest, and I had three sisters; I was the fourth born. We also had an older half-sister who had lived with my paternal grandparents after my father's first wife died during childbirth. My parents are both from the nomadic Bakhtiari tribe in southwestern Iran. Bakhtiaris primarily inhabit Chaharmahal and eastern Khuzestan, Lorestan, Bushehr, and Isfahan provinces. They migrate twice a year with their herds for pasture: in spring to the mountains in their summer quarters (sardsīr or yaylāq), and in autumn to valleys and the plains in their winter quarters (garmsīr or qishlāq).

We grew up in an extended family with a mix of modern and traditional values, both of which were important aspects in my development. In my culture,

DOI: 10.4324/9781003270447-9

the father, mother, children, aunts, and uncles were something akin to a tribe. When a tribe breaks up, so does the family, an experience that can leave one feeling isolated and unanchored.

Before working for the Anglo-Persian Oil Company (APOC) in Khuzestan Province, my father was a journalist and occasional presenter on BBC radio Iran. He was fluent in both spoken and written English. My father's new position at APOC offered him more financial security.

When my siblings and I were primary aged, my mother founded her own school, which she named 'Farah', after Empress Farah Diba, the wife (now widow) of Iran's last Shah, who is currently living in exile in the United States. Many Persians admired Empress Farah in the 1960s; her energy was akin to that of Princess Diana, as was her popularity. In addition to being a fashion icon, she was known for supporting and nurturing artists, including feminist poets and film-makers, and for establishing museums and exhibitions that raised awareness of radical social issues. Farah was also the name my parents chose for me. My mother, who enjoyed making, taught fashion, pattern cutting, and sewing. The majority of those attending her school were professional working women. I started sewing when I was four or five years old, sitting alongside my mother and copying what she was making for us, scaled down in size to fit my dolls.

During the summer in the Khuzestan province, as the heat was unbearable, we would stay indoors in our air-conditioned house with drawn curtains to try to keep cool, spending our time talking and playing together. When the temperature had dropped in the early evening we would go outside to play or stay up late listening to stories told by our elders. In the height of summer, my father would take us to the rural lands owned by my grandparents where we enjoyed the cooler weather and the opportunity to roam freely in the surrounding countryside. In the villages, as if stepping back in time, we observed women spinning wool and dying it with vegetable dyes. The local carpet weavers taught us to weave and we picked our own fruit from the trees. At night, we would listen to the elders' stories. I don't remember ever being bored; on the contrary, I felt the kind of freedom which can only be experienced in childhood when one has no responsibilities or worries. In my memory, it was an idyllic time.

Growing up in Khuzestan, where our extended family lived close by, meant we could see our cousins, aunts, and grandparents regularly and spend long periods of time together. We always had a full house, including the helpers who lived with us. My parents instilled in us the value of being courteous to them emphasising that they weren't there to serve us. We were also taught to respect elders or face consequences if we didn't. I don't recall ever being disrespectful to adults.

Nanne (a term used for mother) Shab Cheragh, who looked after us, dressed in formal tribal attire, with her high cheekbones and imperious bearing. When I first met her, I was terrified of her. But I soon discovered that she was warm and kind and my fear quickly dissipated. My arm has a half-moon birthmark. I recall Nanne Shab Cheragh telling me that my birthmark was a sign of being special and praising me for being a 'good' girl, gently encouraging me not to change my ways ('hichvaght avaz nasho') even when I grew up to be an adult. Her words and powerful presence have stayed with me.

My mother liked to travel and my father's work frequently took him away from home. Nanne was always left in charge and was extremely protective of us. She was also respected by the other helpers who lived with us. She spoke to us in the Bakhtiari tongue, and the stories she told us were ones preserved by an oral tradition, passed down to her through the generations. She usually fell asleep before she'd reached the end which my younger sister and I always waited eagerly for so that we could sneak away to play until we exhausted ourselves and eventually fell into our beds.

My parents socialised frequently; their friends included my father's American and English colleagues. As well as their tribal dialect and customs, both of my parents embraced different art and cultural influences from around the world and a diverse circle of friends including Armenians, Jews, and Baha'is. Although I was too young to be involved in political activities, I absorbed the tension around me. The majority of young people in Khuzestan were drawn to left-wing ideologies, particularly the Marxist–Leninist path to a free Iran. Growing up in Khuzestan province with a large population of Bakhtiaris, there were tensions between the tribe and the monarch dating back to Reza Shah Kabir's (1925–1941) reign as the founder of the Pahlavi monarchy (1925–1979). Succeeding Shahs made concessions to the Bakhtiaris, strategic moves to forestall a toppling of the monarchy in such a delicate, complex political climate.

Moving to Isfahan

When I was nine years old, we moved to Isfahan, a larger city around 400 kilometres south of Tehran, chosen in part because of its significant population of Bakhtiaris. Around that time, my father left the petroleum company. He began to work translating books, films, and catalogues from English to Farsi and vice versa. My parents had decided to build their own home and we lived in a rented house while ours was being erected. I vividly recall regularly accompanying my mother to the construction site so that she could check in with the builders to see how the work was progressing. In order to pay the workmen, we would often stop at the bank first so that she could withdraw large sums of money which she kept in her handbag by her side while driving. I remember being particularly uneasy about the entire process. As I see it now, on an unconscious level, I felt the risks of the situation we were in. On one of the trips from the bank, as our car was about to pull away, two cyclists blocked our path, punched my mother, grabbed her handbag, and took all the cash. Later the boys were found by the police and their family pleaded with my mother for forgiveness. My mother chose not to press charges because they were in their teens and she felt that to do so would have had a disproportionately negative effect on their future. Many years later when I was beginning my career as an artist, I made a series of handbag sculptures, each with either a concealed weapon or with an item to be used in an emergency such as an inflatable life vest. It was a series that had different meanings relating to female identity and societal projections. However, in retrospect, I can see how making these pieces was my way of processing the impact of this very unsettling childhood experience.

In Isfahan, women appeared conservative in their demeanour, with some wearing the Chador, a large piece of cloth like a cloak that is wrapped around the head and upper body leaving only the face exposed. As well, many Mullahs (the honorary title given to Sunni Muslim clergy or mosque leaders), were out on the streets. This was not something I had seen while we were in Khuzestan. I felt discomfort at times when walking with my mother but it was difficult for me to make sense of it because I was so young. My mother didn't wear a head scarf or Chador and instead dressed in fashionable clothing of the time. As we walked through the city, I saw how women were judged based on their appearance and heard as well as felt the comments made about my mother on the streets. She frequently responded to inappropriate remarks made by traditional men with a clever riposte, challenging their views. At the time I wished she would wear a chador so that we wouldn't attract so much attention. Only as an adult did I realise my mother was attractive with her western-style clothing. This, along with the derogatory comments made by passers-by, added to the impression that all eyes were on us. My mother, on the other hand, remained assertive and continued to live in the ways she was accustomed to and had observed with her mother and grandmother. She drove a car, which was unusual in Iran in the early 1970s. She also conversed with the labourers and discussed the work they were doing on our house, a role that was accepted in Khuzestan as the majority were Bakhtiaris and women were accorded high status (Zan Salari) within the tribe. My father, who was frequently away from home, was unable to supervise the building project, allowing my mother to handle it on her own.

There was a significantly sized Jewish community in Isfahan, and my parents had Jewish friends with whom we frequently visited, including over Shabbat. We spent many hours together in their large old house, a place where I always felt comfortable and looked after with a lot of warmth. Iran's Jewish history dates back to late biblical times (mid-1st millennium BC).

The backdrop in Tehran

My recollections, as well as my account of growing up in Iran, are, of course, entirely my own. When, at various stages, my siblings and I have reflected on our home life and childhood years, we've shared similar emotions and perspectives while at other times, not. I am struck by how differently each of us remembers some aspects of our family dynamics, home lives, relationships with our cousins and grandparents, and other experiences from our growing-up years.

Returning to my family's trajectory, we relocated again, this time to Tehran, when I was 11 years old and from thereon we saw even less of our father. It was customary in our culture for the father to financially support or assist the entire family which meant our father worked unusually long hours. I remember missing my father's presence at home and recall him becoming thinner over the years, and even though I was young, I worried about him.

My memories of life in Tehran are of spending less time together as a family and seeing relatives only infrequently. I recall my parents arguing while we were living in Isfahan but I do not remember them telling us that they were separating. As it turned out, they lived apart on and off for many years. We alternated between living at my father's and at my mother's house. I missed my siblings when we weren't together and always felt an internal emptiness when we were separated.

I attended high school in central Tehran from 1973 to 1977. Going to my secondary school, which was near Tehran University, felt a little like being part of a long-running fashion show. We didn't have uniforms and the students, who came from well-to-do professional, westernised families, had the financial means to dress in the latest styles. Many older boys from other high schools and the University congregated in groups in front of my school to socialise. My older sister, who was at the same school, would occasionally take me along with her to meet her university friends. During break times, amongst my peers, we usually talked about current politics and the building tensions which we could all sense. It felt like something was bubbling beneath the surface, and there was uneasiness about being overheard as anyone could be a member of SAVAC, the Shah's secret police and intelligence service in Iran.

My sister was drawn to writers such as Samad Behrangi, a teacher, social activist, critic, and short story writer of Azerbaijani descent. Born into a working-class family, Behrangi was influenced by left-leaning ideologies and a recurring theme in his writings was encouraging the individual to empower themselves to change their circumstances. I was fully aware that his books were banned. If anyone was caught reading or possessing his books, they would be arrested and prosecuted by police. This greatly concerned my parents, who were worried about my sister. The atmosphere in Tehran was very charged as this was the period in the late 1970s, leading up to the 1979 Islamic revolution. During high school break time, we'd hear from older students that even some of our teachers were part of SAVAC and that we had to be careful about what we said. My cousin, who was then a young student and a professional swimmer, was arrested by SAVAC after his family's home was searched for anti-monarchy and left-wing literature. We had no idea what would happen to my cousin and it was a trying time for our entire family. These encounters, as well as my environment, shaped my later consciousness.

My eldest sister, who was in her mid-teens, enjoyed painting and drawing as well as reading and writing poetry. She would frequently talk to me about the poetry of Forugh Farrokhzad, one of her favourite writers, a controversial modernist Iranian poet and film director writing from a female perspective. I remember desperately wanting to understand and to feel the emotions in her poems as I intuitively knew my sister was trying to share with me what she herself was going through. In retrospect, I can see how the poems spoke to her of the agonising and perplexing extremes of emotions that many teenagers, herself included, can struggle with.

Life in England

I left for London in 1977 when I was 15 years old after spending some time convincing my parents that they should send me to the UK to study. The idea came about because a few of my peers moved abroad for this reason and two of my cousins had gone to the United States to further their education. Along with a strong desire to travel, I had carried a sense of otherness which, in part, gave me the impetus to move away from my family and to seek different experiences. I don't recall what I imagined exploring Europe would be like in reality, or maybe I did and now my fantasies from that time have faded, but I was certain that I wanted to leave. What I saw in films as well as the fashionable clothes and the goods sold in the shops in Tehran shaped whatever perceptions I had of England. In my circles, anything imported was accorded higher status. On reflection, most of the serials, films, and musicals that we watched on TV were American, but I hadn't travelled outside of Iran yet, so everything that seemed desirable came from 'the west', a place onto which I unconsciously projected my own associations and meanings. As a young teenager, I remained as quiet and shy as I had been as a child, lacking any of my older sisters' rebellious traits. For this, I was greatly trusted and admired by my parents who saw me as obedient and always made a point of holding me up as a role model to my older siblings, who were more typically adolescent in their behaviour.

Perhaps because of being seen in the family as the 'good child' who was unlikely to get into any trouble, my parents finally relented, agreeing that I could move to England, and my father began the process of determining where I could live and with whom. Studying abroad was, and still is, highly valued in Iran. It was not uncommon for those who were in a position to manage the costs of overseas education and accommodation to support their child in taking up this option. As well, given Iran's expanding international relations, being able to speak fluent English was seen as a real advantage; as a translator, my father placed value on learning the language. In much later years, my oldest sister told me that my father translated films such as *Doctor Zhivago* and *Cat on a Hot Tin Roof*, which surprised me because I knew very little about his work as he never talked about it at home.

My oldest sister accompanied me for a short time but decided to return to Iran because she missed her friends. While she was in London, we both lived with the guardians appointed by my father, a couple with a daughter about my age. They were introduced to my parents by a family friend who split their time between London and Tehran. Our guardians' house was in a quiet London suburb, a stark contrast to living in central Tehran. My parents would call once a week, and I would talk to everyone in my family. We all cried a lot during these phone calls as the extreme distance between Iran and England was now a hard reality, one that often seemed too much for us to bear.

Although always helpful and polite, our guardians seemed somewhat removed and rather aloof, something which didn't have much effect on me until my sister returned to Iran, after which I felt it strongly. I spent a lot of time alone in my room, sad and homesick, missing my family and life in Tehran. During the day, I went to school to study English. In a class of adults from all over the world including India, the Middle East, and Japan, I was the youngest. They were all pleasant and welcoming to me, and, for the most part, I enjoyed being a student. People assumed my family was wealthy because I was Persian, and I was even occasionally asked if my father owned oil wells! However, being away from home was not at all what I expected. The disconnect between what I had imagined and the reality of life in London was extremely disorienting, leaving me feeling displaced and exiled in every way. By contrast, internally I felt rooted and held by my family, with tangible ties to Iran. Eventually I adapted well in my country of exile although I resolved to return home once my English language skills had improved to the point where I could speak it fluently.

Islamic revolution in Iran and the start of the Persian Gulf War

Two years after arriving in London the Islamic Revolution took place. The heavily US-backed and pro-west dynasty of the Shah of Iran, Mohammed Pahlavi, was overthrown and an Islamic republic led by Ayatollah Ruhollah Khomeini was established in its place. Following Ayatollah Khomeini taking power, almost the entire country voted 'yes' in a referendum for the creation of the Islamic Republic of Iran under Khomeini, replacing a monarchy with a theocratic republic, one which the west saw as authoritarian. Overnight, new laws were announced including restrictions on the rights of women, intoducing a dress code that made the wearing of the hijab (head scarf) mandatory.

This was a traumatic time for everyone I knew back home, amplified by the start of the Iran–Iraq war which began a year and a half later. After a long history of border disputes, Iraqi forces managed to take oil-rich Khuzestan, but were quickly repelled and forced out of Iran. Over a million soldiers and a similar number of civilians were killed. Both countries fought until August 20, 1988. Along with the trauma I shared with my family following the revolution, the war brought new pain, worry, and uncertainty about the future. The weekly phone calls with my family, which I looked forward to, abruptly ceased, and contact with them was lost for extended periods of time. Would I ever see my parents, siblings, cousins, and grandparents again? When might the war be over? I felt pangs of guilt, living as I was in a safe place far away from the bombing, interspersed with helplessness, unable to do anything to support them. Through letters from my family and seeing images of Iran on the TV news, I witnessed a seismic change taking place right before my eyes, albeit from afar and filtered through the media. I remember feeling an acute sense of loss and abandonment which I had no one to share with, even if I had been able to find the words to describe what I was going through. I feared for my loved ones as well as for what might happen to Iran, the country of my birth.

I found myself facing a decision to which there was no easy answer: if I returned to Iran, it would be to live in a country that no longer bore any resemblance to my childhood home and my options as a woman would be severely curtailed. If I stayed in London, my contact with my family and extended circle would be limited to visits as and when this was feasible. As this was at a time before affordable international telephone calls, email, or Zoom, choosing to continue my studies in London meant sacrificing more frequent contact with home. In the end, I made the choice of staying in London and enrolled in art school, which is where I began the journey of discovering who I am.

Art gave me a way to get in touch with some of the experiences I had been through including the unexpected severing of ties with my family brought about by long-term involuntary separation. As a form of play, making art draws on unconscious sources and if we can give ourselves over to the process, it can allow us to work through some of our losses and personal traumas. We know the importance of play from psychoanalysts such as Winnicott and more recently, Adam Phillips. In Winnicott's language, "It is in playing and only in playing that the individual child or adult is able to be creative and to use the whole personality, and it is only in being creative that the individual discovers the self" (Winnicott, 1971a, 54).

As Phillips sees it, "for Winnicott playing and reality make each other work, bringing out the best in each other, like a good couple" (2021, 25). Art gave me the opportunity to move back and forth between reality and play, using sculpture, film, photography, and performance to explore and disentangle the strands of my past. In particular, participating in an exhibition mounted by the Institute of International Visual Arts entitled *Veil* which brought together 20 artists and film-makers to examine one of the most powerful symbols in contemporary culture enabled me to better understand what my country had been through in 1979. Artist Marc Garanger, war photographer and soldier during the Algerian War of Independence, was one of the contributors. He had been asked to take identity pictures of Algerian women during the war and the resulting portraits he exhibited are emotive records of the violence and humiliation the women endured, not least, through the act of 'un-veiling' (www.iniva.org). My experience was the polar opposite: I witnessed the loss of many valued personal freedoms when Ayatollah Khomeini came to power bringing in laws which removed the rights of women, including their freedom to dress as they wished. In both Algeria and Iran, the changes introduced were sudden, shocking, and culturally insensitive. Being part of an exhibition project which focused on these complexities and ambiguities, including how they can play out on both personal and global levels over the generations, was a powerful experience for me in different ways. Among other things, it contributed to healing the split I carried, representing the Iran I knew before and after the revolution and the war with Iraq, while also enabling me to own and mourn the losses incurred.

Given my history, it is perhaps no surprise that I ended up training in art psychotherapy and focusing on adolescents. Displacement, and a confused or conflicted sense of one's place in the world, feature in the lives of many of the students I have seen over the years, and not only with those who arrived in the UK from other parts of the globe. I have met young people whose family life was also marked by a significant and abrupt 'culture change,' such as when a step-parent moved in who brought with them different norms and cultural attitudes or when a long-absent father returned, imposing new rules on the family. Adolescents can also be exposed to domestic 'wars' as parents who themselves had little support as children struggle with their unarticulated and undigested pasts, leaving them vulnerable to repeating old patterns or looking to satisfy needs long unmet. Bereavement also creates a sense of 'before' and 'after' of the kind I experienced in losing the Iran of my past. As I see it, my experience of displacement, separation, and loss, although taking place in a very different context and with a degree of economic privilege as a buffer, has given me the emotional and psychological understanding to be able to relate to the clients I see from an internal position of recognition (Akhtar et al., 2020).

If a client is open to engaging in art making, I invite them to do so. This can enable them to represent more painful parts of their experience in a symbolic form as a first step towards being able to name and own it. I too evolved my own art practice in this way, allowing me to 'think with the senses and feel with the mind' (Storr, 2007), an essential quality in any kind of meaningful play as well as in the felt experience of the therapeutic encounter. Being so unexpectedly separated from visiting my family during my adolescence and young adulthood and having to cope with living with strangers is not so far removed from those clients I work with who find themselves taken into care. Although there may be many differences between client and therapist including age and ethnicity, I believe that staying in touch with our own history helps us to better relate to whatever is brought into the room.

References

Akhtar, S., ed. 2020, *Loss: Developmental, Cultural and Clinical Realms*, London and New York: Routledge.

Phillips, A. 2021, *The Cure for Psychoanalysis*, London: Confer Books.

Storr, R. 2007, curator and editor, *Think with the Senses/ Feel with the Mind*, Catalogue published by Biennale di Venezia – Marsilio.

Winnicott, D.W. 1971, *Playing and Reality*, London: Tavistock.

Chapter 9

Holding on tightly, learning to let go

Personal experiences and clinical reflections

Melanie Light

It seems fitting that this chapter is in the middle of the book, not at the beginning. It feels pertinent to my family narrative, which begins before it has begun: family histories which involve fostering and adoption always do. I can recount details about my life in the early 1970s, before my brother came to live with us, but he existed in parallel for some of those years too. I was five and he was two years old when he became part of the family. My early memories are in colour, some hand tinted, some in Technicolour, but without doubt mis-remembered. However, in my mind, and maybe in my brother's, there is an out-of-focus black and white photo quality to his early years. Perhaps there is a relevance to this description, as both colour and black and white have to be woven through our family narrative.

I was born in London into a white middle-class family with a mum and dad and an older brother of 18 months. Shortly after I was born, my mother contracted tuberculosis. My brother went to live with my grandmother and I went to live with my aunt for five months. This was the 1960s when my mother's treatment entailed months away from us in a 'closed hospital'. Her recovery left her adamant that no one, especially a child, should be incarcerated in an institution and led to her decision to adopt a child. Maybe this firmly held conviction had earlier roots, as her own father had been adopted. Or perhaps undetected in the mix was that when my Christian mother married my Jewish father, who was raised in an orthodox Jewish household, he was ostracised by his family.

Once my mother and father decided to adopt, there followed a long process of applications, interviews, and reports, none of which I remember. The first time I think I became aware of anything was at around four years old. We would go and visit a children's home outside London with accommodation for 40 children aged from birth to five years old. Even in the 1970s, residential care was the least desirable option for children in care and the recommended number of children was 12 at most. It was before the idea of key workers and the children were treated in a kindly but efficient manner. Care was done to them, not given. Today the idea of visiting a children's home sounds outdated and makes me feel uncomfortable, but as a child it was what we did.

DOI: 10.4324/9781003270447-10

My parents were asked whether they would consider a mixed heritage child, at that point called 'half caste', and when my parents agreed, the adoption board asked whether they would take a West Indian child and they said yes. This type of adoption is explicitly named now as Interracial adoption or Transracial adoption but I don't remember hearing it then and it was certainly not used in my household. My parents were given pragmatic advice but minimal guidance regarding the emotional experience of adoption and certainly no support in thinking about the complexities of identity and belonging, nor the importance of cultural links and links to heritage this adoption would raise.

When my brother arrived aged two the only thing he owned, his birth name, had been changed in the children's home. His early history was erased yet undeniably hinted at in his skin colour, which stood in stark contrast to that of us, his new family. "The phrase so often used to children being prepared for adoption – the 'forever family' – can easily seem to carry the misleading implication that foreverness stretches both ways: into the past as well as into the future" (Sprince 2008: 107). The past, however far behind in real time, is where the foundation of a child's identity begins, formed from the experience with the parents of their early life: nothing that comes later can replace this. In 1975, Selma Fraiberg introduced the metaphor of 'ghosts in the nursery'. The concept develops the idea that a parent's personal history impacts how they parent their children, a repetition of the past in the present. However rigorous the process of adoption and however much information about the child's early history the parents are given, the implications can be hard to hold in mind. The new parents may wish to forget, ignoring the significance of the ghosts of the original parents, finding themselves unconsciously replicating aspects of that original experience and repeating patterns. The child, likewise, can evoke responses in the adults around them that seem baseless, unless understood as a link to their early history, a haunting by the child's parental figures in mind. As Sprince (2008: 113) suggests, it is vital that "parents fully understand their children's history as well as their child". In the psychoanalytic model of the inner world, experiences from childhood, adolescence and adulthood do not displace earlier ones, but co-exist in the mind, exerting significant influence on later stages of development. So it is vital unconscious memories from the past are understood in the present.

Thirty years later and after having my own three children, I retrained to become a Child and Adolescent Psychotherapist. Informed by my deepening understanding of the significance of early childhood, I allowed myself to be truly curious about the contents of my mind, to reflect upon our family narrative and to think about the unthought. This is not unlike the young people I meet who are at a point where they either *want* to explore, not think at all, or explain away the 'unremembered but unforgotten' (Watts 2001: 18). They may be experiencing inner turbulence, unconsciously re-enacting the psychic consequences of earlier events. They need answers to questions about the past in order to question their future or at least the chance to live more comfortably with these questions. 'Am I the same as other people?' 'Am I weird?' 'Am I different?' They yearn for certainty; however, help is often in the form of being able to tolerate the uncertainty and not knowing. A young person's question is often followed by, 'Do you know what I mean?' because as soon as they've shared something of themselves, anxiety rises and they need 'holding', recognition and reflecting back. Young people need support with establishing their identity, a space to process often complex family circumstances. My work is to think about the infant story held inside, constantly re-enacted in different ways in their current relationships. This requires carefully building a working alliance, receiving the communications, no matter how fragmented, obscure or disordered and bringing them into the 'here and now' of the counselling room to be thought about together. And how much more complicated is this constellation for a child who is fostered or adopted. As Hindle (2008: 17) notes,

> In addition to the loss of the continuity of their lives, many of these children have not had early experiences of attunement and thoughtful emotional interactions that would help them develop the inner resources they would need to make sense of all that happened. For these children, their experiences may be so fragmented and disorganised that it is difficult for them to gather a sufficient sense of who or what has been lost even to grieve.

The door bursts open, Devante, aged 14, recently placed in foster care, arrives with two feet across the threshold of the room, but the rest of her body still leaning outward into the corridor, alerting me to her ambivalence about being here, and perhaps an unconscious fear of allowing herself to settle all in one place. Her face turned towards her friends; she continues her conversation with them. I'm on the end of it, midway through, confused, left out. She beckons them over, "This is Mel", she says in a territorial way, and then looks at me. "I've talked about them before in here, haven't I?", she says conspiratorially. Perhaps we all now know what it feels like to be bit parts and fragments of a story you can't control. The grandiosity she is displaying right now is in sharp contrast to the fragile sense of self she actually holds.

She shuts the door, applies her lip gloss and styles her 'edges' with a comb. ("Edges are the soft wispy baby hairs that grow along your hair line and frame your face. They are the most fragile hairs on your head. It doesn't take much to break them, or pull them from your head." (NaturAllClub.com.blog 2021; NaturAll is a black, woman-owned business.)) Edges are a key part of Devante's look, impacting on whether her day will disintegrate or not. With the recent move to foster care, Devante's 'edges' have got blurred, so she is acting out in school, pushing at the boundaries until she can find some solidity and resistance: a frame.

"I hate it when Miss says I'm not trying. She doesn't know anything! I'm not going to stay in her lesson and be treated like that!" This was a teacher who Devante had warmed to, but now sounded like all the other teachers Devante spoke of – distracted, dismissive, and tired, a mother figure that looks but does not see or validate.

While no one has a positive sense of self all the time, adolescents often see others as perfect or sorted. Adolescence is a time when developmental issues over which they have little or no control come to the fore, but how they pass through these stages can be determined by how they proceeded through infantile development. If a baby receives attuned, interested care giving, they will internalise a sense of being intrinsically interesting. As Winnicott (1971: 134) states, "When I look, I am seen, so I exist". Having a sense of your own self-worth means not having to act upon your anxieties or fears that you are unworthy, unlovable or invisible. Gerhardt (2009: 10) suggests, "It is as babies that we first feel and learn what to do with our feelings, when we start to organise our experience in a way that will affect our later behaviour and thinking capacities". A relationship built on pleasurable interactions is essential to regulation and the building of a self-image, which impacts our expectations of others and how they will behave and which in turn influences how we feel about ourselves. Gerhardt goes on to say,

> Most parents instinctively provide enough attention and sensitivity to their baby's emotional security. But what seems to be most crucial for the baby is the extent to which the parent or caregiver is emotionally present and available, to notice his signals and to regulate his states.
>
> (2009: 21)

Often the young people I meet, like Devante, have had parents who have been unpredictable or emotionally unavailable to them, leaving them with an inability to think about, and therefore regulate themselves. They are stuck, feel overwhelmed, and their 'self-esteem' is adversely affected. The therapeutic work begins with a process of listening, of being curious and wanting to think about who they are and who they can become. If the young person hasn't experienced this in their earlier lives, it is another chance to become understandable and to be understood. We are relational beings who emerge and organise ourselves in engagement with other live minds. Peter Fonagy (2003) refers to the brain itself as a 'social organ'. In the earliest weeks and months, we need someone to respond to us, without too much anxiety, to comfort and regulate us, building our capacity to trust that the world is a reliable place. Only then can we safely become physically and psychologically separate beings. We need enough dependency in order to become independent.

Kelis, aged ten, had experienced profound neglect and had witnessed domestic violence and was now living with a maternal aunt. In sessions, she liked to play school, where she cast me as the teacher and she had the role of the permanently-first-day-at-school student. Most of the game took place in the imaginary foyer of the school. Kelis would wait to be collected for her first day, alerting me to what it felt like to be alone, yet still with the hope of being found and reclaimed. The student in the game always wore the wrong uniform, perhaps highlighting the feeling she didn't belong anywhere. Notably, the student had more knowledge than all the other students in the class; perhaps a way of letting me know she knew more than most children should. In the game Kelis would constantly break rules and be sent back to the foyer ashamed and unclaimed, unable to belong to the new class/family. In Sibling Matters, Smallbone (2014: 190) notes, "children whose family life is disrupted to the extent that they are received into care suffer great disjuncture and trauma to their sense of stability and safety". The game was repeated weekly for months until Kelis was able to become the teacher, and I the student. As the teacher, she was terrifyingly tyrannical and often sadistic in her demands, but it seemed to relieve something within her. She had a chance to be in control as the authoritarian adult, and as the student I was able to ask questions of the terrifying adult figure. This game helped Kelis metabolise her experiences and put into words some of what she had felt and seen, all the while staying safely in the metaphor.

Rustin (2006: 17) identifies a fundamental question for children who are fostered or adopted: "Where do I belong?" She points out that "(t)he idea of belonging somewhere is an ordinary and fundamental building block of personal identity". To safely be an individual, children first need to feel contained and identify with a well-functioning family. The sense of belonging brings additional developmental challenges for looked-after and adopted children, whose sense of identification, being valued and noticed may not have been securely established previously. Parker (2020: 39) identifies further questions: "Who do we identify with? Who do we wish to emulate? Who is on our side?... Who feels different? We need parental recognition and appreciation, but arguably being valued and noticed by our siblings matters even more".

Two years after my brother came to live in our family my sister was born, so now there were four of us. It gets tricky at this point because if I have to describe the make-up of my family, I say I have an older brother, an adopted brother and then get into words like 'a real sister' or a 'natural sister' – somehow suggesting my brother is abnormal or unnatural. It upsets me! What I do remember is how strongly my mother encouraged us to find the glue between us, to hold on to each other very tightly. Thinking about these times makes me reflect on sibling relationships and the ongoing impact they have on how we make sense of ourselves, the people around us and the groups we do and don't form. Siblings are the longest-lasting of all family ties, and in my case, sibling relationships will probably survive much longer than my parents who took the decision to adopt. Parker (2020: 5) states,

> Relationships between siblings are constantly shifting emotionally too, swinging between huge ranges of experiences.... all these sibling

experiences form a blueprint, shaping the way we respond to competition and cooperation, the assumptions we make about others, and the type of relationships we form.

My mother called us WARM – an acronym of our names that bound us close and I think at points left others out in the cold. There were reasons for keeping us close, perhaps more so than in other families, because we were visibly different. Our family's way of creating belonging was through love overcoming difference and positively pursuing colour blindness. I grew up with no concept of a racial identity. Certainly up until secondary school, my family were in the mainstream and we had a mono-racial upbringing. The issue of difference was marginalised; there was no attempt to meet the contradictions or duality of my brother's everyday life. Our parents were very thinking and engaged people, yet at that time, there was no 'requirement' or 'advantage' in thinking about how to support him to develop a positive black racial identity, which would be vital for his self-esteem and a sense of who he was. In my lifetime there has been a shift in adoption practice which previously viewed black children as 'unadoptable' or 'hard to place' (Small, 1982; Rowe, 1991). A critique emerged that cited agency failure and institutional racism as the main causes of the shortfall of black families (Kirton, 2000). However, our family was growing up in Britain in the 1970s and 80s. Painful feelings of 'you don't belong' ran like a refrain through our childhood. Jackie Kay, the author of Red Dust Road, who was an adopted black child of a white, Scottish couple, in a similar time period, writes of how people of colour were constantly told they didn't belong and the impact this had.

> It is not so much being black in a white country means that people don't accept you as, say Scottish; it is that being black in a white country makes you a stranger to yourself. It is not the foreigner without; it is the foreigner within that is interesting … Children have an intense need to belong and anything that marks them out as different from all the other children will then form a straggly queue of uneasy, queasy questions in their head.
>
> (2011: 38)

When I undertook my psychotherapy training, I initially struggled in thinking about difference, unpicking it, or even realising it had to be acknowledged. It felt like a denouncement of the position my family had actively taken and fought so hard to maintain. From training onwards, I have had to confront issues of belonging, physical and cultural dislocation, the impact of racism, and my complicit part in upholding this. I am still very much a work in progress. Perlita Harris (2006) addresses the realities for black and minority ethnic children of being raised by a white adoptive family, in a collection of testimonies called In Search of Belonging: Reflections by Transracially Adopted People, "noting the extra complexities around allegiance with British culture and Britain, the importance of names, lack of history, coping with questions from others, inter-nalised racism, self-hate, body image and emotional distress". I have to carefully examine my own narrative and the subjective phenomena which shape my pres-ence in the counselling room. In a large London multi-cultural school, I have to check my identification with and availability for the young people with whom I work. I must constantly address my own and the collective cultural blind spots, acknowledging and examining a racist backdrop to our society, which although I had believed I was not part of, I now realise as a white person I could not be free from.

Like individuals, families tell autobiographical stories too. 'Hold each other tightly' was my family story. The story functions as a mirror, similar to the mirroring of a baby from birth, when it looks to its mother for confirmation of its existence. Do I recognise myself in this family story? If you look and see something unrecognisable, anxiety is stirred up. In cases of adoption the mirroring process may well be distorted. In an attempt to integrate both the young person's reality and their fantasy, questions arise. 'Who were my first parents? What were they like? Why did they give me up?' These are questions that may not be obviously voiced, because adoption can often be about things unspoken, but are rather interwoven throughout their material and there to be heard.

Tyrone, aged 17 and adopted at birth, talks about his now ex-girlfriend; "I just want to see her one last time. I want to ask her why she let me go. Why has she abandoned me? I feel like I'm an outline with a big question mark in-side". These could be questions meant for his birth mother. Mehmet, aged 14, adopted at two years old, arrives at the session in disbelief. He has been going out with Frankie for two months, "She dumped me on my birthday!" he shouts, standing and angrily slamming the lid of my bin down and kicking it. "I took the sweatshirt she'd given me and stuffed it in the bin right in front of her". Mehmet's feelings about his 'birth' day are alive in the room. Our task was to sit together and grapple with the anger and humiliation felt in the here and now and then at some point approach the original hurt. As he stiffly bent down to pick up the bin, I wondered whether he could experience me as offering a containing function for the powerful primitive anxieties he wanted to dump. Could he safely express the rubbish parts of himself in here? Could I bear wit-ness to his pain, to see him, and perhaps in time leave him feeling less like an 'outline?' For "self-esteem is not just thinking well of oneself in the abstract; it is a capacity to respond to life's challenges" (Gerhardt 2009: 89).

According to Calvocoressi and Ludlam (2008: 185):

> The psychological process of belonging and becoming encompasses two profoundly important and linked developmental tasks. In belonging, we form attachments to others with whom we identify. They become our kith and kin. Once a kinship attachment has been formed, we can embark on becoming, the process of establishing a sense of self and identity.

One way families do this is by naming each other's similarities; young people's identities begin to form from what they see and hear from others, comments like, 'He's just like me; I was no good at maths either' and 'she has her mum's sense of humour'. In combination with the ways we imagine others see us, we create stories about ourselves and these form our core beliefs, both positive and negative.

Young people who have experienced trauma make assumptions about being no good and believe that is why they have endured the experiences they have been through, however irrational this way of thinking is. 'If my boyfriend dumps me', the automatic thought is 'I am unlovable'. Similarly, 'I did badly in that test' becomes 'I have no value'. The reaction to the hurt is amplified and punitive with no sense of balance.

Establishing a sense of identity and developing a better understanding of complex family circumstances are interlinking processes. Adoption adds further complexities such as issues of identity, questions to do with origins, loss, sense of self and belonging. These span both the inner and the outer world and are intimately linked with the relationship to the self and others. Put another way, an adopted young person will have

> in mind a version – more or less conscious – of what their birth mother and father felt about the loss of their child. This may be the product of imaginative conjecture, or what the child has been told, or a combination of the two. However it is arrived at, it is likely to have a significant influence on the child's sense of self and self-image; that is, whether the child imagines the birth mother and father felt sadness at the loss of their child, or relief, or indifference, or – worst of all – felt glad to be rid of them.
>
> (Hindle, Shulman 2008: 5)

A sense of belonging comes from meaningfully resembling someone, reflecting the biological and psychological link to the birth parents. Whilst most children can look at their parents and see current resemblances and even anticipate how they might look as an adult, an adopted child has to create a parent first who resembles themselves, whom the child in turn can resemble before the developmental task of individuating can take place – a task linked to establishing a secure identity.

Jackson, aged 7, knew nothing about his parents and had been placed in care when he was young. He played in our weekly sessions with the Spiderman action figure, which compelled me to look up the back story of Spiderman:

> Peter Benjamin Parker is an orphan living with his Uncle Ben and Aunt May …. he is bitten by a radioactivespider … Along with heightened athletic abilities, Parker gains the ability to adhere to walls and ceilings … and fire adhesive webbing.
>
> https://en.wikipedia.org/wiki/Spider-Man

Through his play Jackson was letting me know something of his internal world. He would fire string from his Spiderman and wind it round my hands, literally making a physical attachment to me. Soon he included the doll's house in his play. The doll's house had a detachable staircase and at first he left it in the box. A solitary plastic figure would sit silently on the second floor of the doll's house, waiting to be rescued. Spiderman would sometimes come to the rescue if he wasn't too busy saving the world, and the two would talk to each other and share pretend food. Later, Jackson began to attach the staircase to the doll's house and Spiderman would walk up, rather than fly in. Eventually the Spiderman figure was replaced by another 'more normal' plastic figure and the good friends, as they had now become, were free to come and go as they pleased. While I was not part of the game play, I would act like a gentle voice-over to the action, the way a mother might, regulating the baby's feelings, entering the baby's state, validating the baby's experience. My sense was the sessions gave Jackson a chance to be in touch with a listening other, which helped him develop a more objective picture of who he was: neither superhero nor voiceless victim. He acquired a sense of his own agency and efficacy.

My work in schools means I spend lots of time with young people who are in an ongoing dialogue with themselves. They need someone to recognise and respond to them. As Nick Luxmoore (2008: 22) notes: "Our separate existence, our sense of self depends paradoxically on other people understanding how we feel and what we want". All psychotherapy involves this, but with adopted children the adoption has to be kept in mind too. This involves recognising each child's individual trauma and dysregulated state holistically, in order to re-ceive, to tolerate and then slowly to name it. "The naming allows thought about why something happened, to enable a coherent narrative to be constructed, so that meaning can be discerned and emotions processed and thought about" (Hindle 2014: 251). Or as Bion (1965) put it: The *what* has to precede the *why* or the *how* of any emotional experience.

Lauren, 15, had been living with foster parents for a number of years and had sporadic contact with her birth mother. "My mum lives nearby, but she wouldn't recognise me!" she declared in an offhand manner. Lauren had been in trouble in school that day. A supply teacher had told her "You've done no work!" at which Lauren erupted, getting herself sent out of class. For Lauren it seemed to have translated into "You're not worth anything". Her brittle sense of self felt annihilated. Without the initial experience of regulation, young people struggle to regulate their own feelings. In schools however there are absolute regulations, from morning registration to the bell at the end of the day which are further reinforced through detentions and exclusions. Lauren would be given a detention for being sent out. Once a little time had passed and I had listened and heard what Lauren needed hearing in that moment, we thought to-gether about whom the supply teacher might remind her of as a teacher coming and going and only taking an intermittent interest in her. We recognised she hadn't had the mum she deserved and there would always be a disappointment in looking for a mother who might never be able to *recognise* her. This was real, this was unfair. In future sessions, we took time to think about our relationship and the regulations that came with it, including our ending, and all the mixed feelings that we would need to discuss, "But not today, Miss!"

Whatever the reason for a child being separated from their original family, it will leave scars. There may be a limited experience of early regulation, which encompasses a baby's basic responses being elaborated and developed into more explicit and complex feelings. Rebecca, age 11, had been adopted aged four, as her mother had experienced mental health issues and drug dependency. In one session Rebecca was sticking strips of Sellotape in straight lines onto paper. For her, sticking and gluing seemed to be a way of attempting to explore the threat of fragmentation: how we hold ourselves together, who 'sticks around' and how we keep ourselves attached. She was attempting to get a pipe cleaner to stick to the paper, but it kept pinging off. "It seems like a difficult job to get anything to stick today", I offered. "Yes, it is!" She asked for PVA glue, a ruler, and tracing paper – none of which I had. I was beginning to feel like an ill-equipped, unprepared mother. "It must feel like I can't give you what you want. That must be frustrating". She looked at me sideways and nodded. She began to cut a heart to stick on but was beginning to get annoyed, as each time she tried to cut the shape, the scissors cut too deeply and jaggedly. She looked at me, "Can you fix my heart?" I felt truly moved and said, "Let's work together to fix it. You hold the paper and I'll cut gently round it". We continued, with me commenting on what we were doing, using a calming tone of voice and non-verbal cues, to help get Rebecca back to a place where she felt comfortable again. When it was time to leave Rebecca stuck a googly eye on her hand. "Perhaps with that stuck on your hand, it feels like I can keep an eye on you when you're not here". She laughed joyously. For Rebecca, learning to trust was hard and today she needed something physical to take with her. Winnicott (1951) spoke of transitional objects as bordering the child's early fusion with mother and their dawning awareness of separateness. A particular object can be used as a way of regulating fears of being separate or alone. The object is the representation of the child's internal unity with a nurturing, adaptive mother. Growth and development imply a linear age and stage progression; however, there is constant oscillation and interplay between ever-shifting states of mind. Today, Rebecca, who was still developing the capacity to internalise a mothering figure, needed a transitional object – something from the session to stick with.

My brothers and sisters have stuck together and are still very close with a WhatsApp group called WARM. My brother (I still resist calling him 'adopted') continues to find it hard to say goodbye on the phone and I tend to have to be the one to say it. Every ending is difficult, forever resonating with the original ending.

We are confronted by endings all the time when working in schools, from the end of each lesson to half terms and holidays, the end of each school year and the final one coming at the end of full-time education. I sometimes end work with a child because it fits in with school terms, or else they may be leaving for secondary school. There are a lot of goodbyes. Can they ever really be *good* byes? I know I have struggled when the therapy ends, handing the children and young people back to make their own way in the world. It is an area I have worked on many times in supervision. Adoption hopes to offer a happy ending: "a way of alleviating distress – recompensing the children for their previous lack of a happy family life, giving them the kind of family they should have had from the start" (Sprince 2008: 102). In my clinical work, I have learnt there is no such thing as a perfect ending, just the aim for something good enough and as Jackie Kay (2011: 45) writes, "You think adoption is a story which has an end. But the point about it is that it has no end. It keeps changing its ending".

Casey, 11, had been living with her mum's long-term partner. Her mother, a known substance abuser, came and went. During the time we worked together, Casey was placed with a short-term foster carer. Our work came to an end when Casey moved on to secondary school. The whole of her last term in Year 6 had been about her *not* coming to therapy; she began each session by saying she wouldn't stay, but once in the room she remained for the entire time. In the final session, Casey went through her art folder, but only took things that were A4 size, unconsciously giving me what was too big to manage and also leaving something of herself behind. She was distracted and the room felt rather like the morning after a party: a bit hopeless and empty. She seemed awkward and looked dismissively round the room, her gaze finally landing on a pile of books in the corner. She picked one up, opened it and held it directly in front of her face. I, too, now felt hopeless and empty confronted by a visible barrier that seemed hard to penetrate. I sat quietly, hearing her breathing and slowed my breath down, until we were in sync. As I sat, the significance of the book's title, 'What Happened to the Dinosaurs?: A Book About Extinction' struck me. Casey had found a way to acknowledge the ending which, perhaps until that moment, we were both finding too painful to address. Carefully commenting on the title, I thought aloud about the 'extinction' of our physical sessions, noting how I felt sad about the ending, but how I would be able to remember our time together. Rather than the sessions becoming 'fossilised', perhaps Casey would be able to hear my voice when she needed to think something through. She lowered the book and nodded thoughtfully, looking at my face intently. It was a moment of genuine connection; I knew something of the sessions would remain preserved in her internal landscape. She then snapped the book shut, almost visibly putting her body armour back on, ready to go back to class.

In his poem entitled 'Inspire and Be Inspired' Lemn Sissay (2015), also a fostered child, implores us to let go of our defences and foster an open mind, one which researches and questions, embracing all our dreams. Perhaps someday in the future, Casey will be able to put aside her 'armour' more often in relationships, feeling more at ease in letting her spontaneity and enjoyment shine through.

My brother is my brother is my brother. Do I still believe that love is the most important thing? I absolutely do. If you love and share and breathe and grieve as a family, it matters. Do I feel there could have been a more thought-through way of him understanding his background and owning and being proud of his heritage? I absolutely do. Pivotal life events have of course contributed to my personal and professional functioning and the theoretical position I take. My clinical technique continues to be shaped by ongoing, imperative, and enriching understanding. My family taught me how to hold on tightly, and I continue to learn and trust in letting go. For the young people I 'hold' for a while, I hope to offer a chance to open the door together with them, often very slowly, sometimes having it bang shut unexpectedly but being ready, when the young person is, to ask, 'What was it closed for?' To be alongside them to think about the questions and the answers, before letting them go, to get on with getting on.

References

A. P. Carter; Luisa Gerstein Cups Song Songwriter(s): Pitch Perfect 2012 Production Company Gold Circle Films, Brownstone Productions.

Beth Hall and Gail Steinberg (2013) *Inside Transracial Adoption* London and Philadelphia: Jessica Kingsley Publishers p. 17.

Debbie Hindle and Graham Shulman et al. (2008) *The Emotional Experience of Adoption - a Psychoanalytic Perspective* London: Routledge.

Debbie Hindle and Susan Sherwin-White et al. (2014) *Sibling Matters -a Psychoanalytical, Developmental and Systemic Approach* London: Karnac p. 251.

Derek Kirton (2000) *'Race' Ethnicity and Adoption* Buckingham: Open University Press.

Donald Winnicott (1951) *Playing and Reality. Transitional Objects and Transitional Phenomena* London: Routledge.

Donald Winnicott (1971) *Playing & Reality Mirror-Role of Mother and Family in Child Development* London: Tavistock Publications.

Doug Watt (2001) Emotion and Consciousness: Implications of Affective Neuroscience for Extended Reticular Thalamic Activating Systems Theories of Consciousness' www.phil.vt.edu/ASSC/watt/default html

Francesca Calvocoressi and Molly Ludlam (2008) *Shared Reflections on Parallel Collaborative Work with Adoptive Families* in *The Emotional Experience of Adoption - A Psychoanalytic Perspective* London: Routledge pp. 205–212.

Jane Rowe (1991) *An Historical Perspective on Adoption and the Role of Voluntary Agencies* in Joan Fratter, Jane Rowe, David Sapsford and June Thornburn (eds) *Permanent Family Placement: A Decade of Experience* London: BAAF.

Jackie Kay (2011) *Red Dust Road* London: Pan MacMillan.

Jenny Sprince (2000) *The Network Around Adoption. The Forever Family and the Ghosts of the Dispossessed* in *The Emotional Experience of Adoption a Psychoanalytical Perspective* London: Routledge (2008).

John Small (1986) *Transracial Placements: Conflicts and Contradictions* in Shama Ahmed, Juliet Cheetham and John Small (eds) *Social Work with Black Children and their Families* London: Batsford/BAAF.

Lemn Sissay (2015) A poem from University of Manchester's Lemn Sissay to commemorate his installation as Chancellor.

Margaret Rustin (2006) *Where Do I Belong? Dilemmas for Children and Adolescents Who Have Been Brought up in Long Term Foster Care*, in Jenny Kenrick, Caroline Lindsey and Lorraine Tollemach (eds) *Creating New Families: Therapeutic Approaches to Fostering, Adoption and Kinship Care* London: Karnac.

Margaret Smallbone (2014) *Brothers and Sisters in Care* in Debbie Hindle and Susan Sherwin-White (eds) *Sibling Matters: A Psychoanalytical, Developmental and Systemic Approach* London: Karnac pp. 190–205.

Nick Luxmoore (2008) *Feeling Like Crap: Young People and the Meaning of Self Esteem* London: Jessica Kingsley Publishers.

Nick Luxmoore (2019) *The Art of working with Anxious, Antagonistic Adolescents* London and Philadelphia: Jessica Kingsley.

Perlita Harris (2006) *In Search of Belonging: Reflections by Transracially Adopted People* BAAF.

Peter Fonagy (2003) The Development of Psychopathology from Infancy to Adulthood: The Mysterious Unfolding of Disturbance in Time *Infant Mental Health Journal* 24 (3): 212–239.

Selma Fraiberg, Edna Adelson, and Vivian Shapiro (1975) Ghosts in the Nursery: A Psychoanalytic Approach to the Problem of Impaired Infant-mother Relationships *Journal of the American Academy Child Psychiatrist* 14: 387–422.

Sue Gerhardt (2009) *Why Love Matters* how affection shapes a baby's brain Routledge, https://naturallclub.com/blogs/the-naturall-club-blog/how-to-grow-back-protect-and-maintain-your-edges, https://en.wikipedia.org/wiki/Spider-Man.

Val Parker (2020) *A Group-Analytic Exploration of the Sibling Matrix - How Siblings Shape Our Lives* London: Val Parker Routledge.

Chapter 10

Masculinity and the male therapist

The internal and external struggles

David Trevatt

Introduction

One of my earliest memories of being at school in the 1950s was when we were each told to make a picture of the union flag on paper. These pictures were then stuck on little poles for parading outside in the playground on what was called 'Empire Day', celebrating the colonisation by Britain of approximately 171 countries and 25% of the land surface of the world. As a young child I assumed this was the natural order of things and something to be proud of.

In my childhood I regularly read about the British army defeating the cowardly Germans or the Japanese and watched 'westerns' featuring the defeat of the indigenous populations of North America and thought little about it, except that 'we' were better, braver, and the winners.

The mythology of the victor still persists in our culture, making it complicated to have a balanced view of our heritage when the truth of our role in the world is so sanitised. We were the upholders of honour and decency, creators of the 'mother of parliaments', and a democracy that was the envy of the world where other countries were depicted as the purveyors of false images of themselves.

Once I moved into adolescence I came not only to question these received truths but beyond that, to believe that we had much to account and atone for. I still feel it is not possible for me to uphold the many achievements that this country has made over centuries without acknowledging the truth of the more shameful acts perpetrated in our name.

Growing up in post-war Britain

These were turbulent years in this country and abroad in the form of civil unrest, strikes, conflicts, and anti-war protests uniting disparate groups such as students and workers, religious leaders, and intellectuals. There was a spirit of revolution and liberation; of questioning and often rejecting the norms of the established adult order in favour of a counterculture that challenged what was considered outdated values and repressive institutions; rather like the process of adolescence itself.

DOI: 10.4324/9781003270447-11

In my late teens I became curious and interested in the opinions of others, often getting involved in discussions late into the night. Being able to argue and express personal opinions and hear others was a pleasure, even when some opinions were radically different to my own, indicating that I had a lot to learn coming as I was from a relatively sheltered and privileged suburban background. Studying psychology and sociology opened my eyes and my mind even more to what was out there, but also to what was in there – in the mind.

The concept and practice of communicating feelings became highly important to me, partly because I saw this as something I needed to improve in myself. I came from a family and culture where the 'stiff upper lip' approach to expressing feelings, particularly amongst boys and men, was encouraged. I came to understand this as a defence against vulnerability and being seen as weak. Feelings kept buttoned up signified control and mastery of oneself and projected an image of strength. However, we know from research evidence that low emotional expression is frequently a contributory factor in poor mental health, including serious mental illness (Leff, 1985). Distancing oneself from personal feelings has enabled men in particular to engage in the horrors of warfare for centuries.

The adolescent task

Adolescence can be a time of re-evaluation, of no longer accepting the values that are imparted by the adult world. This was certainly my experience. Young people are confronted with many tasks, amongst which are the personal, physical, and psychological changes that they experience in this tumultuous development phase. A great many questions are in play about the self: 'where am I going?', 'what will become of me?', 'how will my life unfold?', 'what do I need to survive?' to name just a few.

The adolescent begins to critically evaluate the adult world and their own burgeoning place in it. In the process of moving towards adulthood themselves, they have the opportunity to use their new-found range of feelings and perspectives to find their own voice, their own mind, and opinions.

Among my memories of adolescence was the strength of feeling and passionate belief I had in issues such as social justice, with an acute sense of unfairness as for many of my generation. Life for some appeared settled and comfortable, bringing with those privileges the potential for power while for others it was hard, discriminatory, and devoid of choices.

My family had working-class roots and my generation was the first to become broadly middle class. There were no clear expectations beyond 'doing one's best' and attaining a good average and my experience of formal education was less than positive. When school was not boring it was terrifying. Some teachers were kind, encouraging, and even inspiring, but I experienced many as sadistic, prone to belittling and scornful remarks. Violence by staff on children was commonplace and accepted; child-on-child violence was equally so.

Conformity was demanded and self-expression was not encouraged. Friendships were important, if not vital.

Despite all the difficulties to navigate during my schooling, I was keenly aware of the 'gateway' function of education, how it could lead to opportunities and greater freedoms in life, and that without doing well in examinations those possibilities became closed off.

Through my own experience of adolescence and later, through my work with young people, I came to realise just how fundamental the building of confidence and self-worth are: qualities that can only be achieved through succeeding in something. I had my own experience of struggling with self-doubt, diffidence and failure mixed in part with success. This motivated me in later professional work to become involved in supporting young people encountering these common difficulties.

In my therapeutic work in schools I have encountered many young people who struggle with the feelings that failure – or the fear of it – has brought to them, leaving them feeling marginalised, under-achieving, depressed, angry, and hopeless: feelings that can endure for a lifetime if unprocessed.

I saw first-hand during my years of work in social care before embarking on psychotherapy training the extent to which disaffected young people can become oppositional and defiant in the face of the demands of teachers, parents, and the wider world. From the data and from our own empirical experience, we know how disengagement with education can not only lead to disruptive and destructive behaviour by young people but can also affect those around them. From the perspective of the disaffected, education exists for the benefit and glorification of schools and parents, not for them. They may set themselves against any efforts to help them in the belief that there is more to life than qualifications.

Learning about people and the self

I graduated in social sciences during the 1970s and during that time I found myself challenged in many different ways including personally and politically. It was a troubled decade with many strong voices and opinions abounding. I found my way into social work where there seemed to be many people who cared about the disadvantaged including children, elderly, mentally ill, physically disabled, and ethnic minorities. Social work was mostly undertaken by women; I had several inspirational female colleagues and supervisors and felt comfortable in this environment although male roles and societal prejudices against women were frequently and vocally challenged.

I was exposed to a range of people with needs and a political context for meeting those needs. I also began an association with the Tavistock Clinic which was in the borough I worked for. I sought out specialist supervision which helped me deepen my understanding of the problems I was meeting in my work. This led initially to various training courses for social workers, from where I moved into personal psychoanalysis and culminated in a very long and complicated training in child psychotherapy. I learnt that there is an inner world which is not governed by the same underpinnings as the external world. But more importantly I learnt about the place of the emotions in defining who we are and how feelings motivate the individual as well as wider communities and nations. I came to understand how they are fundamental to how we behave, how we react and how we understand – or misunderstand – ourselves and others and therefore the extent to which they bear further scrutiny.

Training in child and adolescent psychotherapy

Why train in psychotherapy? What is the link between the outside world – a reality that can be filled with such beauty and such horrors – to the inside, where we barely perceive what is going on? I think the connection is that, knowing there are such terrible examples of human behaviour throughout history, we can try and understand what drives some people to these acts, whether against a child, an adult, a community, a nation or an ethnic group.

I remember in some long-ago training session being invited to reflect on what made us decide to become a therapist from the context of our family of origin, looking at special circumstances that might have led us to choose this career. Factors may include the position in one's family or social group or being situated somewhere on the periphery, given to observing rather than being immersed in it. In reflecting on my family experience, I see myself as being the awkward one who 'would not be told', questioning rules and demands made by my parents. I was seen as obstinate and difficult. I was annoyingly analytical at that age of adolescence where refusal and challenging instructions were not welcome but somehow irresistible. 'Why are things the way they are?' 'Who says so?' I was known for taking oppositional views to established ones and being drawn to supporting the underdog in any dispute. My brother, who is three years older, had to give way to me as the reliable, responsible one at a young age while I could enjoy the protected space he allowed me to have. But where he conformed I did not. Where he met expectations, I was something of a disappointment, making my own way in a rather haphazard fashion, looking for something different.

As for most if not all of us, my option to study human behaviour through psychotherapy was not unrelated to the position I had in my family. Psychotherapy or psychoanalysis offers the opportunity for us to understand, confront or accept certain features of ourselves. This doesn't mean that the opportunity is actually taken. I remember hearing during training that some people can undergo years of analysis without being significantly affected or benefitting from it. Therapists may be in this position too. We have all encountered therapists who prefer to attend to the problems of others rather than look too closely at themselves.

But in the normal circumstances being a therapist draws us into an exploration of the self and from there, the mental states of others. This leads to deeper understanding, facilitated by the therapeutic relationship. Having said that, we all have unconscious processes at work and in addition we may have 'blind spots', things we may choose not to see or know about or be impervious to aspects of ourselves in the way that others see us.

Learning to be a man

My experience of being male in what has historically been referred to as 'a man's world' has meant I have had to reflect on my own prejudices and preferences as well as the wider question of what men stand for in a society privileging males. This was certainly the case as an undergraduate and also in radical social work, where men were in a minority and challenged in their traditional roles as protectors and leaders within the family and in the wider world.

Expectations of boys can be considerable, even when their ability to exercise authority may be limited. I have encountered times when the man is looked to for guidance or explanation because of their gender rather than having any particular ability. It is within this prevailing culture of routine sexism and misogyny that adolescent boys grow up, often driven impulsively to externalise their strong emotions, sometimes with little thought or regard for others, particularly girls and women. Helping them to identify and understand what these emotional impulses are and where they come from is fundamental, especially when they may have had little guidance from fathers who themselves struggle with masculinity and are distant, uninvolved, or absent.

Learning from the adolescent

I avoided working with adolescents for a long time. Perhaps I saw them as too difficult, or not far enough away from my own experience to be bearable; too confused and confusing – and too annoying. Having faced these objections during psychotherapy training I frequently confronted the reality that adolescents referred for therapy did not always engage, possibly because it was not their idea in the first place but rather the wish of a parent or teacher. Unlike younger children, adolescents are quite capable of exercising their will by not turning up if they do not want to, particularly when it's to a service that clearly has the label of 'mental health' attached to it. Even in schools where the psychotherapy service is more available and more acceptable as 'counselling', it can be regarded as shameful or demeaning. I have seen young people being persuaded by others not to enter the therapy room in school because it is not the thing to be seen to be doing. This is where recent increases in community-based therapy services, where peer exposure isn't an issue, can be a more effective base for adolescents to use.

Learning from the disturbed adolescent

On the understanding that we learn more from our failures than our successes, my first experience as a child psychotherapist provides ample material. Twelve-year-old Jonathan was my first psychotherapy training patient whom I was to see three times a week for at least a year, an apparently pleasant teenage boy from a prosperous family. His parents had separated after his father had started an affair with the family nanny who subsequently had a child, a younger brother for my patient. Jonathan lived principally with his father following the divorce and remarriage. His behaviour became more and more difficult as he was shunted back and forth between his parents, who ran out of patience with him. His father, a strict disciplinarian, resorted at times to physical punishment. The family hoped that therapy would help the boy calm down and accept the new family circumstances.

It was clear that Jonathan felt unwanted and in the way. He was aggrieved but unwilling to talk about these feelings in his therapy and any attempt to encourage this met with great resistance and an aggressive response. He felt that his therapy was punishment for his existence and that everyone would happily carry on with their lives if he was no longer there.

He tried to bargain his way out of therapy, becoming more oppositional and challenging in his sessions. He played around with the boundaries, arriving late or absenting himself entirely. He would throw stones at the windows from outside and once inside the building he would run off around the clinic gleefully bursting into occupied therapy rooms. His fantasies became more aggressive and violent. He brought out pornographic pictures from his bag, masturbated, and urinated in the waste basket. He would throw himself at me from the window ledge like a young child so that I had to catch him to prevent him from hurting himself. And he accused me of being a Nazi concentration camp guard who had killed his family.

I attempted to contain his excessive behaviour. When I called a halt to the therapy sessions, he pleaded with me not to stop or tell his father how he had behaved. I was caught between dragging him back to the waiting room or giving him another chance to behave in the therapy room. He resisted interpretations of his actions as his regressive behaviour increased and hated any suggestion of sympathy, attacking me all the more in a bid to deny his vulnerability. I felt my main task was to survive these sessions: to not give up or give in, to not rise to provocation and retaliation, and to remain kind and thoughtful even if this was not welcomed.

From time to time Jonathan would have momentary Kleinian 'depressive' interludes where another reality intruded to replace his paranoid-schizoid attacks. For example, he reflected on what he might want to do when he was grown up, "Maybe I could be something cool like a therapist". He fantasised about the family life I had and envied what he thought it was like. At times he seemed exhausted by his oppositional attacks and showed a different side where he appreciated me and my role with him. In the transference I was often a hated figure, but then he would overcome his rivalry, accepting his desire for an affectionate relationship. I thought he very much wished to be close to his father, as if seeking both 'punishment and reconciliation', feeling both 'admiration and envy' (Salzberger-Wittenberg 1970).

Somehow we both survived the experience for over a year (at three times a week!) but his behaviour at school and at home was deteriorating and he stopped coming to therapy. I heard from his father that he had been sent off to boarding school. There had been no ending for the therapy, no period of drawing to a close. I was simply presented with the fact of his relocation.

I can't emphasise enough the importance of my supervision and personal psychoanalysis in helping me to withstand this year-long experience of degradation. Fuelled by emotional pain, he had become adept at communicating his feelings directly and non-verbally, giving me the experience of how he felt inside: broken, furious, and inconsolable.

Jonathan turned up unannounced several years later to see me at the clinic. He appeared quite a subdued young man, presenting as friendly and approachable. He asked me if it would be possible to continue his therapy with me, saying he could not remember much about his time with me before but he thought he might not have treated me very well. I had to tell him I could not continue to work with him because I was leaving the clinic. He accepted my explanation without question. I was interested that he came to see me and that I had remained a 'good object' in his mind in spite of what we had been through. I was also pleased to see that he seemed to be relatively at peace with himself as a young adult.

In classic psychoanalytic theory the Oedipus complex is thought to occur in boys and girls throughout their development but is felt more keenly during adolescence when rivalries with the same-sex parents and desire for the opposite-sex parent are consciously and unconsciously enacted (Klein 1959). Without both parents being able to offer containment and understanding of these developmental issues the adolescent can be left unable to process their identity development and sense of self. I felt that Jonathan had encountered the break-up of his parents traumatically, feeling unwanted by both of them, and this is what he brought to therapy and enacted within the safe structure provided.

I wonder what this experience might have been like for a female therapist. Would he have been so out of control and violent? I have seen several boys with quite severe levels of emotional deprivation as well as victims of severe physical and sexual abuse, boys who have formed a strong attachment to me but at times have violently acted out. Often the abuser is a man. Therefore the male therapist is frequently confronted with the full force of the rage against and fear of the abuser in the negative transference that develops. The abuse, it appears, results in psychosis being projected into the child.

Feelings evoked for or against the adolescent in the therapeutic work are important to take into account, especially where emotions often run very high. In working with young people we may feel provoked to anger, boredom, sympathy, fear, or distaste. We can't like everyone, nor should we try to but we can identify and reflect on the feelings that they stir inside us. Again, supervision can be invaluable in creating some perspective in the frequently fraught relationships that might entail deep loathing or love, attraction or repulsion. It can help us untangle the knots we may have become embroiled in. With Jonathan I was left trying to encapsulate the essence of the issue again and again through interpretation, while repeatedly being buffeted by his projections of inadequacy. I recognised his attempts to behave so badly that I would reject him and this strengthened my determination not to give in or give up.

Working in schools and the institutional transference

Further into my training I took over as a school-based psychotherapist in a boarding school for boys with emotional and behavioural difficulties. It was a job that no one else wanted at a tough school. On arrival I was greeted by the school secretary who, in a loud cheerful voice, announced: "Oh you're the new school psycho!..."

Many of the boys I saw there were very guarded and distant with me; one even asked me nervously if I could read minds. This all said something about how both the staff and students felt about themselves as well as how they thought they were seen by the outside world and, ultimately, how I might see them.

The atmosphere in the school was defensive: physical punishment was sometimes used by staff against the violent attacks of the pupils, and pupils retaliated verbally. Damage to the school was frequent. Windows were regularly smashed, making the local glazier a regular visitor. I could certainly understand the staff's frustration with the destructive behaviours. Equally I could understand the mammoth uphill struggle to enable these boys to accept and trust anything 'good' in others or in themselves. They were the bad kids sent off into the middle of the country, far from their homes and communities. They had personal histories of family breakdown as well as physical, emotional, and sexual abuse. They tested the emotional patience of staff to the limit and further, unearthing the anger and humiliation beyond the friendly offers of help and support. Many staff needed space to recover their composure after engaging in the daily battle of wills, where their professional selves were regularly taunted and twisted and threatened.

Psychotherapy offered a radical respite from the battlefield that the school dynamics often resembled. On one occasion, in a group I ran for some of the older boys who were leaving at the end of the school year, several attendees were playing up, sabotaging the sessions as they often did, moving one boy to ask in frustration "can't we just *talk*?" It was a telling remark: talking and thinking were things that most of these boys tried to avoid as much as possible.

It brought to mind Bion's distinction between thoughts and thinking. Thoughts occur naturally but the activity of thinking requires a certain environment:

> If the patient cannot "think" with his thoughts, that is to say that he has thoughts but lacks the apparatus of "thinking" which enables him to use

his thoughts, to think them as it were, the first result is an intensification of frustration because thought that should make it "possible for the mental apparatus to support increased tension during a delay in the process of discharge" is lacking.

(Bion, 1962)

Working in a school for children with severe physical disabilities provided a different but allied context. There were few behaviour problems here, and none of an extreme nature. The atmosphere of the schools was bright, positive, and cheerful, very much focussed on what young people *could* rather than could not do. Young people had to contend with life-limiting conditions, undergoing repeated operations to correct or ameliorate severe illnesses. They often had complex needs and used imaginative forms of communication to express their immediate needs for help with going to the toilet, eating, breathing, epileptic seizures as well as their feelings. Staff were very attentive, warm and in tune with their needs and able to anticipate many of them by the way they vocalised, looked, or gestured.

As the school-based psychotherapist, I was seeing these young people who were also undergoing the normal processes of adolescence. Some parents found it hard to allow their sons and daughters much freedom because of a desire to shelter them like much younger children which was driven in part by the anxiety that they would get into difficulty. So therapy was a place where some of these young people's wishes and frustrations to become independent could be aired and explored. This could be made more difficult by their ways of communicating or their struggles to use speech, where words might be few and hard to arrange in a way that made sense and yet were often full of meaning and emotion. They presented a pressing desire to be taken seriously as a young adult rather than treated as a dependent 'child' whose body did not function like able-bodied people's.

On one occasion a teenage girl came to see me and said she wanted me to help her stick paper over the window in the door of the therapy room which led out into the main school corridor to provide privacy. The head teacher informed me afterwards that the paper screen should be taken down as it was school policy for all rooms to be open for observation from outside. I accepted this ruling but wondered about the girl's wish for privacy in an environment where there was little of it. The physical needs of the majority in such a school dictated the requirement for constant supervision. I think that there could have been a concern about a teenage girl seeing a male therapist without supervision being available. In a way this checking is a protection for the male therapist not to be compromised or be left open to allegations of misconduct, which is a constant consideration in working with young people in distress or poor mental health. Indeed, I worked with many sexually abused girls (and boys) who were overtly disinhibited or sexually provocative. My parameters were very clear and strictly adhered to: firstly, to use supervision to monitor and manage such cases.

Secondly, to ensure provocative behaviour is managed in the session by an open narrative interpretation of events i.e., articulating what the child may be attempting to do or show by their behaviour. Thirdly, by kind yet firm limits, including minimal or no physical contact so that there is no misunderstanding of the relationship between patient and therapist.

Working with the parents of adolescents

There are still many adolescents today who won't attend sessions in any setting. We know that the recognition of having a mental health problem and then doing something about it, such as seeing a professional, indicates a degree of health through showing motivation. Adults as well as young people can feel embarrassed by the idea of having a mental health problem and will go into denial as a defence against thinking, feeling, and taking action.

This points to the importance of services aimed at supporting the parents of adolescents who are unwilling to engage with help on their own behalf. Parents are often the only adults their reluctant or withdrawn adolescents are in contact with and are often optimally placed to help their adolescent children; they know them best and are the most committed to them. But they themselves need help in knowing how to understand and respond to their adolescent's needs. To this end, therapists can work with the adolescent through the parent, providing specialist help indirectly to the adolescent as well as directly to the parent.

In my work with parents of adolescents I frequently came across parents who had strong beliefs that their child should have the right to experience freedom that they themselves had not enjoyed when they were young. Sometimes this approach has led to the adolescent not having the necessary structures and limit-setting that would enable them to feel contained. I've often observed that rather than bringing happiness to the adolescent, unlimited freedom resulted in a more demanding and critical attitude towards their parents and others precisely because of failing to provide boundary-keeping and limit-setting.

I remember seeing the parents of an adolescent girl who, when sent to her room as a punishment for staying out late with older friends, would escape through her bedroom window to continue her socialising outside. When she subsequently got into trouble she complained to her parents, "Why didn't you stop me?" One way of understanding this is that she wanted her parents to stop her from her own wayward impulses when she could not stop herself.

Parents of adolescents can often feel frustrated for not 'getting it right'. They feel as if they are wrong either by being too strict and therefore authoritarian, or too indulgent and libertarian. The result is a double negative: they blame themselves and are blamed by their child. This can be further complicated when adolescents use their understanding of their parents' strengths and weaknesses to play them off against each other to their own advantage.

Male psychotherapists engaged in parent work can be helpful in supporting mothers who may be isolated or do not have access to male parental influence in the parenting of their adolescent. The issues of parenting young people who are undergoing complex changes require considerable thought and reflection, ideally by both parents in order to respond appropriately and adequately. Male psychotherapists may be able to assist through some modelling that can help fathers to respond to adolescents in ways that offer constructive alternatives to withdrawing, rejecting or giving way to anger or harsh criticism. What is needed is a calm and strong authority (in an often highly emotionally charged environment) that fosters the acquisition of the adolescent's own nascent authority and their ability to think for themselves. It is hard work to find a balance and it requires constant review and adjustment as the adolescent matures. Because the therapist is focused on promoting the parents' own sense of expertise, it's crucial that we hold our consultative role and be alerted to any idealisation of the 'expert' coming from the parents.

Conclusion

Traditionally, not many men have trained as child psychotherapists. Most of the teaching staff when I trained were women and there was perhaps an assumption that working with children was more of a female preserve, where women had more direct experience and interest than men.

There is a clear need for more men to enter the profession. Male psychotherapists have the potential to bring something useful and different to young people in therapy. Along with female child psychotherapists they can foster a nurturing role for adolescent minds and together with parents can demonstrate a present, active, and functioning figure. They also can provide a model that may be missing in the lives of those young people who have grown up without a present, consistent, and secure male figure.

Many women, mothers, girls, and boys have had negative experiences of men. One does not have to look very far to find prominent examples of male behaviour that are destructive, violent, demeaning, offensive, and abusive, or just absent through abandonment of the family. Such absence can be personally felt by each child as somehow their own fault for not being good or lovable enough for the father to stay. How essential is it then that there are trustworthy, reliable, kind, and safe alternative examples of men available?

I never make assumptions about what I, as a man, represent to people in therapy. I understand that it may take a long time, if ever, to be trusted when someone has been severely let down or has suffered injury or harm at the hands of a man in their life. Why should they take the risk of trusting a man, even if he calls himself a psychotherapist, who may betray that trust?

This in some ways explains the severe testing and challenging by abused boys and girls that male therapists are often faced with in different ways. Sometimes the child is withdrawn and fearful, sometimes flirtatious and seductive. "What kind of a man are you?" they seem to be saying, "You appear okay on the surface but what about underneath? If I challenge you in this way or that, will you reveal your true self and turn out to be the monster I suspect you might be?"

Young people have much to defend and to protest against. The world is a dangerous place. Children, young people, and women are right to be cautious about trusting men who may not be worthy of it. In such a climate as we find ourselves in, the need for male therapists who follow the codes of decency, truthfulness and respectfulness is as pressing as it ever has been.

References

Bion, Wilfred R. *Learning from Experience* p.84 Maresfield William Heinemann Books Ltd, London 1962.

Klein, Melanie 'Our Adult World and Its Roots in Infancy' p.252, (1959) In: *Envy and Gratitude and Other Works 1946–1963* Hogarth Press, London 1975.

Leff, Julian 'The Concept of Expressed Emotion: New Empirical Evidence' pp.501–509 In: Pichot, P., Berner, P., Wolf, R., Thau, K. (eds.) *Epidemiology and Community Psychiatry* Springer, Boston, MA 1985.

Salzberger-Wittenberg, Isca (ed.) 'Anxieties Related to Loss and Mourning' p.103 In: *Psycho-Analytic Insights and Relationships: A Kleinian Approach* Routledge and Kegan Paul 1970.

Chapter 11

Suspended animation

A traumatic family history without a context

Gwendolyn Rowlands

Introduction

The killing of George Floyd in May 2020 saw a resurgence of the Black Lives Matter movement sparking global protests and leading many individuals and organisations to pledge to address long-overdue racial inequalities. As an art psychotherapist who works with children and adolescents in schools, I joined a peer group whose focus was on how we might engage with issues around race and the dynamics of the therapeutic relationship as well as wider issues of inequality, both personally and professionally.

Reading the book *Me and White Supremacy* brought to my awareness the extent to which the legacy of the transatlantic slave trade persists, with its structures still present in all aspects of our lives today (Saad, 2020). Saad's assertion, which I agree with, is that we live in a society that is set up to allow a smooth path and multiple benefits for one group of people at the expense of another; and that because of this each member of society must take responsibility for racial inequalities. Once I started to notice white privilege in one area of life it was possible to begin to see it everywhere and I found myself in agreement with her.

Given that I had always considered myself a liberal anti-racist I was shocked by the complacency that the book confronts the reader with. Saad (Ibid) and Diangelo (2019) note that the shame induced by recognising white privilege often results in 'white fragility'. As someone of Anglo-German background this premise had particular resonance for me. It led me to the question of whether it is ever possible to atone for the past? Most of my life has been spent with an awareness of the Holocaust. But to compare the two – the Holocaust and attitudes to the past in post-war Germany and white responsibility for societal racism faced by Black people and those of colour today – seemed at best confusing and at worst highly inappropriate. But this is exactly what Susan Nieman (2020) looks at in her book on the subject.

Neiman's unique perspective has illuminated my family history and changes in post-war German society that I was completely unaware of. A distinguished philosopher who comes from a Jewish family from Berlin, her grandparents

DOI: 10.4324/9781003270447-12

had fled the Holocaust. She grew up in the southern United States where she witnessed extreme racism which, while principally targeted at Black people and those of colour, also extended to Jews and other minorities. She subsequently moved to Berlin to take up an academic post in the 1980s giving her deep insights into Germany's attempts to deal with the legacy of the Holocaust.

During my art psychotherapy training there was insufficient time devoted to cultural competency for it to be explored in depth in spite of it being an essential element of all counselling and psychotherapy courses. But as with all areas of professional development, training is just the start of an ongoing process spanning our professional lives. My personal struggle to understand a complex family background and the ways in which it had impacted me continues to be a crucial component in my development as a therapist: in all aspects of therapeutic training we start from the self. In areas where we have good self-understanding we are more able to make ourselves available for our clients. So it followed that opening up to the complex themes of racism and identity raised questions in my mind about my own background that had not been fully explored or resolved. In engaging with anti-racism, the only place to start was with myself and my family's history. In this way my focus shifted from contemporary issues of racism and colour to the racism represented by the Holocaust. The link was taking personal responsibility for understanding the past and my family's role in it but none of this would mean anything unless it translated into becoming more aware of current inequalities personally and professionally and developing strategies for addressing them.

My story

I was born at the tail end of the generation whose parents directly experienced the Second World War. With a German mother and a British father my family was caught between two sides of the conflict. My mother came to the UK in her early twenties, six years after the end of the war, and was classified as an Enemy Alien. She was required to report to her local police station long after her marriage to my father until she became a naturalised British subject. My mother chose total assimilation including a complete mastery of the English language so that no one would know that she was German. Unconsciously she may have felt she had no choice but to immerse herself in the studious application of British custom and culture, but on the other hand she adored everything English and thought of England as a spiritual home. Both my parents came from humble beginnings and rose high in life by reconstructing their identities to enable themselves to fit in. This gave them a certain vulnerability to setbacks along the way, and at times they ran the risk of being shamefully 'found out'. Would my mother have made such an uncomfortable choice, coming to the UK so soon after the war, had she not been a 'looked after' child?

My mother was orphaned when she was seven years old after which she went into long-term foster care. She came from a poor working-class family. Her new foster family were from a higher social class that had, before the war, been able to afford servants. My mother had many happy memories of her family of origin and the sense of being different from her new family. At times her foster mother would emphasise that she had come 'from the gutter' which did not fit in with her own sense of pride in her origins. It was in this context that my mother's departure for a new land might be understood. She had nothing to lose and much to gain by finding her own place where she could truly become herself and if she did face a struggle to fit in, that was nothing new to her.

I grew up with hidden differences and in the first three decades of my life it was not uncommon to hear people openly express their hatred of Germans. Behind this attitude lay stories of a father, uncle or brother who had never returned home from the war. There was an ingrained hatred borne out of the propaganda and privations of two world wars, but beyond this was the certainty that the British had the moral high ground and had held strong against an evil regime. Central to post-war British identity was a hard-won victory that took everything the nation had. Echoes of it endure to this day through references such as 'we'll meet again', a World War II song that became a reassuring talisman through a different crisis, most recently in the 'fight' against an invisible 'enemy' during the first lockdown of the pandemic. Growing up in the 70s in this country, my experience of British national triumphalism contrasted with the self-confident modernity of the post-war German 'economic miracle'. Behind both myths lay some uncomfortable truths: on the British side, about having won the war and lost the peace. On the German side, it was about an economic success that allowed that society to enjoy prosperity and high status while at the same time masking its new identity as a defeated, occupied and divided country.

My childhood was spent in suburban London, the youngest of three children in a white middle-class family in which we all went to the local state primary school. Somehow the other children got hold of the fact that we were half-German. In the playground the children taunted me and called me 'Nazi' and I would come home and ask my mum if we were 'bad'. As Neiman (2020) puts it 'Evil' is what others do. Our people are always very fine people.

Growing up I came to live with the idea, as my mother had done before me, that other people would not like *my* people as they had done a very bad thing indeed. My mother, a natural storyteller, recognised the value of sharing her history and was willing to answer my questions regarding the past unlike those children of trauma victims who find themselves faced by a wall of silence. However oral history is partial and what is left out can be as important as what is relayed. In putting together this account I have become conscious of the themes these stories captured. Why was a particular story told and what was its real agenda? As an adult, I have come to question these narratives as though hearing them for the first time.

Back then, my mother was able to unfold the family story in a simple, age-appropriate way and over the years of my childhood the story was repeated in greater detail. Each time it was recounted my understanding grew and new questions were asked. Now, long past childhood, reviewing these tales I see that they contain the notion of 'goodies' and 'baddies' that needed to be confronted. But this also spoke of my inability as an adult to deal with the shadow of a trauma as big as the Holocaust. Seeing her own children grow up and reach the age at which she experienced so many traumatic events must have triggered in my mother the need to tell her childhood story and to attempt to process her unresolved grief and trauma. When I was eight, I wanted to know if my family had done 'something bad' and, if so, how this fitted in with my upbringing, which placed emphasis on knowing the difference between right and wrong. I needed to understand more about Hitler and what it was like for my mother growing up in the Third Reich, what my grandparents and foster grandparents had done, and how the German people could have been taken in by such an evil man.

My mother was born in Germany. She was orphaned in 1939 at the start of the Second World War when she was seven years old. Like large numbers of unemployed working-class people in the 1930s, her parents died of illness brought on by poverty. This led to being placed in long-term foster care; she was not adopted and kept her birth family's surname. Although contact with her birth siblings was limited, she managed to stay in touch with all five of them throughout her life. My mother's foster parents were highly educated people who took my mother in out of a sense of religious duty. They raised and educated her with love and care and saw to her every need but were unable to provide the physical warmth and affection of her own more emotionally demonstrative parents. My mother stored up every memory of her birth parents and idealised them. They were forever perfect in her internal world.

My mother was seven at the start of the war and 13 years old at the end. Her war-time experiences would have been similar to those of a British child from a big city. There was the impact of aerial bombardment: terrifying nights spent in air raid shelters, the interruption to education, the loss of their home; the front was blown off my grandparents' apartment, the loss of friends and neighbours killed in bombing raids. Eventually, she was evacuated with her foster mother and foster brother. They went to stay in a small village in the Westerwald region. The area was Catholic and it took the villagers a while to accept my protestant family. My mother spent mornings at school and afternoons working in the fields. There she and her fellow workers (women and children) were subject to repeated aerial attacks. Their only recourse was to lay flat in the open field.

Unlike her British counterparts she found herself in the midst of the German retreat that marked the end of the land war, on the western front, in mainland Europe. By the end of the war Germany was in a state of total collapse and this coincided with two hard winters in '46 and '47. Many people starved and many without homes for shelter froze to death. My grandmother did not talk much about the war, but there were frequent references to going hungry. She would say things such as, "we prayed for food and it arrived". Many of my mother's stories featured going hungry and somehow food arriving from unlikely sources. I grew up with a superabundance of food and as a small child, I was overfed in reaction to these experiences. The consequence for me was being overweight as a child and as an adult, the lingering habit remains of not being able to leave any uneaten food on my plate. Like many children of previous generations I was made to sit indefinitely at the table until I'd cleared my plate.

Arguably the biggest trauma for my mother was not the war but being orphaned and the ongoing consequences of that loss. Her five siblings were scattered and during the war it must have been unbearable not knowing where they were, and whether they were safe. In 1945 the whole of Europe was on the move with people returning from the war. In addition, there were many displaced Germans and German refugees flooding in from former German-occupied countries. In towns and cities small handwritten notices were put up on walls as people sought lost family members. It was at this time that my mother's 15-year-old brother miraculously appeared in the village with nowhere to go. As an apprentice engineer, he had been evacuated with his company to do war work and fend for himself. However, my mother's foster parents declined to take him as he would have been another mouth to feed. Heartrendingly, my mother accompanied him as far as she could on his onward journey before returning home.

In 1969 when I was five, I visited Germany for the first time. The visit lasted six weeks – the extent of the school holidays – and during this trip we went, with my Oma (German for grandmother), to visit the Westerwald community where my mother had been evacuated during the war. In preparation for my first trip abroad, I was taught to pack a suitcase and told that, from hereon, this was my responsibility, something which triggered anxiety that I see now had a deeper source. During the holiday I ended up in hospital with a severe tummy ache with no discernible cause. Looking back, I think it is likely that I absorbed my mother's childhood history which of course would've come to the surface during this visit to Germany and was, no doubt, unconsciously projected onto me.

Aged eight, I asked my parents if I could join the Brownies, a question they took very seriously. My mother explained that around the same age, she had been forced to join the Hitler Youth which left her with feelings difficult to reconcile about the Scout movement (which included the Brownies for girls). I was invited to make my own decision perhaps replicating my mother's childhood experiences of being given important choices with moral implications; doubtless she took this as the norm. With somewhat mixed feelings, I joined and, to their credit, my parents both supported me in taking part.

My mother's foster father, my Opa (grandfather) was an academic who taught at the university. A philologist, he specialised in the study of ancient Greek with its associations to the New Testament and Hebrew with its links to the Old Testament. After Hitler took power in 1933 the influence of the National

Socialists took over every sphere of life including academia, and in order to teach at a German University you needed to be a party member. My grandfather refused. As a young child I learned this as a fact, but I could not start to comprehend what this act of resistance would have meant for him and my family. To refuse to join the party generally meant either death or being sent to a labour camp. All I knew was that he had survived.

My grandfather was already in his forties at the start of the war. Many of his students were Jewish and in the preceding years had, one by one, started to disappear from his classes. My mother told stories of the Gestapo coming to their door when he was at work to frighten him into compliance. They were frequently terrorised in this way. As the war started and more men were conscripted, Opa took over preaching in a Lutheran parish that had lost its pastor to military service. His sermons were prepared in duplicate and a copy of the text was handed to the Gestapo sitting at the back of the congregation. He could not afford any misunderstandings. But it seemed the regime had other plans for him. Opa's knowledge of Hebrew put him in a vulnerable position. The regime used his scholarship opportunistically, forcing him to catalogue the many Jewish books including those that came from private collections confiscated by the Nazis when their owners were sent to concentration camps. This must have been a hideous perversion of everything that he valued, a form of psychological torture. Accepting this form of work would have meant the difference between life and death for him and for the rest of the family too. But by accepting such work the authorities had made him complicit in their evil.

Any study of the Third Reich shows that there was no effective opposition to the Nazi regime. This included the Catholic and Protestant churches in Germany. The regime took over the Lutheran church erasing all references to the Old Testament that would have linked it to the Jewish faith. However, my family belonged to a dissident religious group that refused Nazification, known as the Confessing Church. Its most well-known member was Dietrich Bonhoeffer, vicar, and theologian who took part in a failed attempt to assassinate Hitler for which he was imprisoned and later executed. Another prominent member was the theologian Martin Niemoller who wrote the oft-quoted poem entitled 'First they came…' which poignantly highlights the cost of not speaking out when individuals are targeted because of their beliefs or their identity. It ends with the chilling observation that, if we fail to stand up for others, there will be no one to speak out for us.

Niemoller became one of the leaders of the post-war Lutheran church. The first Lutheran church synod after the war, attended by my Opa, made a public declaration of collective responsibility for the regime and the Holocaust, known as the Stuttgart Declaration (Marcuse, 2005). I was told this as a child: this responsibility was central to our Christianity. As an adult, I understand that it does not matter who my family were or what they had done: that we *all* hold responsibility along with the rest of the German people for the evils of the Third Reich and the Holocaust.

It is difficult for me to accept the past and I can recall the many ways in which I continued to deflect my attention away from it. Like most young children, I held in mind an absolute binary between good and evil. In my childhood, I accepted the family stories as they were presented to me. Unable at that early age to understand the nuances or implications, I concluded that my mother's family were indeed 'good people'. I was reassured by the fact that there was nobody old enough in my biological family to have fought in the war. My mother's birth parents lived until 1939 leaving them potentially enough time for political engagement but although I cannot know for certain, it is unlikely as they were preoccupied with struggling to survive. And in my mother's extended foster family? One uncle was a field surgeon on the Western Front, and also a member of the Confessing Church. Another, a cousin, was executed by the Russians in reprisals for German atrocities. As the only single person present without spouse or children, he volunteered to take the bullet. I could kid myself that, really, the war and the Holocaust had nothing to do with me or my family, that somehow as dissenters we shared in the guilt but were on an entirely different moral plain, a view that could never hold. An aunt by marriage showed me a photo of her much-loved father, dressed in Nazi uniform. I had not even thought that most families would have had someone of that generation in uniform however it did not alter my perception that the war and the Holocaust did not have anything to do with my family. I was shocked when, staying with a family friend as a teenager, I spotted to my horror a framed photo of my host as a young man in Nazi uniform and next to it his iron cross. He did not attempt to conceal that he was an unrepentant Nazi. If anything these events served to reinforce the idea in me that the German side of my family was significantly different to and' better than' other German families.

Feeling different

The ongoing exploration of who I am in the context of my family narrative has had a strong influence on my therapeutic work with children and young people. Along with enhancing my understanding of the complexities of multiple identities, it has opened my thinking to the effects of others' assumptions of who we are based on nationality, ethnicity, and the colour of our skin.

A 13-year-old pupil I worked with, Zana, was anxious and depressed. She used her sessions to try and work out how she was feeling. As she became familiar with the therapeutic process and what counselling sessions could offer her, she became able to access some difficult emotions. Part of what emerged were questions about her identity and how she fitted in with her peer group. In an attempt to alleviate her depression, she told me that her mother had suggested that she pray to Allah. She said, with feeling, "People don't think that I am Muslim, but I am". As part of an ethnic Albanian Kosovar community her family had settled in the UK after the war in the 1990s. It was not part of her culture to wear a headscarf and she looked European, especially as she was surround by girls in her class who did wear headscarves. She had become an invisible Muslim. What assumptions were being made about her and what impact was this having upon her? I commented that as Islam is a world-wide religion, wondering what she thought a Muslim might look like. But this was beside the point and didn't address her feeling of difference. Her discomfort was compounded a few weeks later when she reported that her family had been subjected to an act of racism, as she described it, simply because they had a foreign-sounding surname. Her parents were silent about the past and its traumas. A trip 'home' during the school holidays found her mother in tears mourning Zana's grandfather whose death remained unexplained to her.

In the diverse and mobile population of the UK today dual or multiple identities are commonplace. But our sense of self may in part be dependent upon what stories we feel able to tell about ourselves and our forebears. For many people it is the struggle to find a mirror of their own family narrative in the wider culture that disrupts their sense of self.

My parents separated in the mid-1970s and I did not see my father between the ages of 11 and 18. I then became cut off from the English side of my family, which was small to start with. In the school holidays I was packed off to Germany to stay with relatives and so spent more time there. My parents' divorce had a huge impact; at that time it was not as common as it is today. I felt singled out at school and let down by my parents who had taught me that divorce was against our religion. I was angry and started to see hypocrisy everywhere, including in the Church of England, the state church of the country to which my parents belonged. Studying politics at A Level raised my awareness of the British constitution and the links between the government, church, monarchy, judiciary, and the military. This was during the cold war and I questioned how a Christian church could promote war; I came to the conclusion that it was immoral. I joined several peace groups and spent my spare time on demos and trips to 'embrace the base' at Greenham Common with other women anti-nuclear protesters. I also campaigned with friends on green issues like removing lead from petrol. I was evangelical which annoyed my peers at school who would not see things my way. I was horrified by their apathy.

To my surprise, my activism served as a catalyst for my strict old-fashioned grandmother to begin sharing stories with me about *her* peace activism. She came from Strasbourg, a border city and grew up fluent in French and German. At the start of the First World War in 1914 her German family was forced to flee to Germany. As a young woman in the 1920s she became a supporter of the League of Nations, the precursor to the United Nations. After the Second World War and well into her 1980s she became a member of the peace group at her church.

I had a long-held fantasy that had I grown up in Germany, somehow I would have been better equipped to process the legacy of the Holocaust. In German there is a word that refers to the decades-long process through which Germany has started to come to terms with Nazism and the Holocaust: *Vergangenheitsaufarbeitung*, which literally means the struggle to overcome or work through the past. For me, the experience of being Anglo-German has cut me off from this discourse.

This in large part helps explain the centrality that my sense of being an outsider has to my identity. Growing up as an Anglo German I could not see my background and experience reflected in the culture surrounding me; there was no context to help me understand where I belonged. In the first three decades of my life there were only occasional glimpses that allowed me to make a connection to who I was. The underlying contradiction I felt beset by was that I live and I am at home in one culture which expresses most of my values and shared ideas. However, there is another part of me that on the one hand holds the familiarity and the intimacy of my mother, but on the other, is distant and unavailable through geography, history, and my own limited language skills. Nor does any word exist to describe this contradiction, this intimate alienation. These factors are a significant aspect of my background that have gone on to shape and inform my work with young clients who are in some way caught up in complex family histories.

Growing up I was cut off from the discourse in German society regarding the legacy of the war and the Holocaust. Unlike most Germans my mother was open about what had happened to our family and was actively engaged in telling our stories and helping us to make sense of the past. She had come from a family that encouraged engagement in moral questions and growing up she had been required to take on board such things. On the one hand I learned about the Holocaust and my family's role in it. On the other, I had no way of contextualising it and setting it alongside other German family stories. There was no sense of how these might differ or converge. My family seemed to be a one-off. When we went to Germany such things were not discussed, or if they were I had no access to them as I wasn't brought up bilingual. Growing up I got on with being a 'normal' English person while having this hidden story as part of my heritage that was too significant to ignore.

Neiman (2000) plots the course of post-war German society from its immediate aftermath, which was dominated by a complete denial by ordinary Germans that they were in any way to blame for the Holocaust. Kahn (2020) notes that the local residents of the town next to the Dachau concentration camp had wanted to bulldoze the camp in the 1950s after an influx of visitors who came to see it. Denied that possibility by the regional government the town instead opted for something subtler: it took down the street signs that pointed visitors to the concentration camp (Hammerich et al., 2016).

In 1968 the student protests that took place around the world took their own shape and form in Germany. In the USA the focus of the protest was against the Vietnam War and the start of the civil rights movement. The need by the student protestors to call authority to account held a particular significance in Germany. Almost everything in politics and society was called into question; not one area of life was spared critical scrutiny. In the 1960s and into the 1970s information began to seep out about atrocities committed during the Third Reich by the parents of the 1968 generation. Many of those individuals had moved smoothly into positions of power in the post-war period. The Jewish author Ralph Giordano calls this 'the second guilt'.

> Any second guilt presumes a first – in this case, the guilt of the Germans under Hitler. The second guilt: the suppression and denial of the first after 1945. It has significantly influenced the political culture of the Federal Republic of Germany until today – a mortgage that will take a long time to repay.
>
> (Giordano, 1987)

The parents who were 'the silent generation' gave way to their children of 'the raging generation'. Battle was openly declared against this 'second guilt' – against duplicity and hypocrisy at all levels of society. With hindsight this bitter struggle for a better society and a protest against the silent paralysed parents was the struggle to maintain an intact ego ideal that united both generations and became a solidarity of silence about the evil and murderous past. The perpetrator's children became inwardly indivisible from their parents: on the one hand they developed the narcissistic ego ideal that the parents had lost and on the other, they functioned as a cruel and punishing super ego when these ideals were not realised (Hammerich et al., 2016). Neiman (2020) records the incredulity she experiences from those outside Germany at the degree of the German people's denial of the Holocaust and how they cast blame elsewhere. While she understands the depth of German people's suffering during the war and in the immediate aftermath, in no way does she excuse their denial.

In thinking about my own story, I have relied upon the writing of Prophecy Coles whose study of intergenerational trauma shows the importance of the lives of previous generations within families and how trauma is passed down the generations. She looks at the lives of the children and grandchildren of Holocaust survivors and how this trauma continues from one generation to the next. But to find myself to any extent in this I have drawn upon the work of Hammerich et al. (2016) which focuses on dialogue between second-generation perpetrators and survivors of the Holocaust. The work of Kaslow (2000) further documents experiential group work by survivors and perpetrators run over a number of years by the American Family Therapy Association.

There is a family story that seems to sum up so much that cannot be said in any other way. During the war Opa would take the train home on leave on leave to where my family was evacuated. On one journey he fell into conversation with a monk which was interrupted when the signal was given that they were under attack and must disembark. Opa tried to give his coat to the monk whose white robes would have made him a target but he refused to take it and Opa said, "Then I cannot stay with you". The story underscores the tensions in my grandfather's life. He was neither a saint nor a Nazi. He risked his own life by refusing to join the party, he left his church when he saw that it had been utterly corrupted and joined a dissident church. And while he made the decision to save his life and that of his family by accepting work that involved complicity with an evil regime, he was amongst the first to publicly declare corporate responsibility for the evils of the Third Reich. Although out of step with the state of denial adopted by the vast majority of German society in the immediate post-war period, the judgment by history passed on him and dissenters like him was that this was too little, too late.

My sense of *Vergangenheitsaufarbeitung* continues as I try to work out the past. In 1933, 30,000 Jews lived in my mother's home city. By the end of the war only 602 remained. As I grew up I understood that the well-kept villas that we had passed on the way to the children's playground in my grandparent's neighbourhood had once been the homes of Jewish people. In contrast, after the war Opa resumed his professional life, returning to the University and continuing to correspond with friends and colleagues abroad who managed to get away.

Piecing together the stories from my past and trying to understand the nuances and implications of my German heritage has, and continues to be, a lifelong task. For those of German heritage, issues of identity and self-image are particularly complicated. It was not my intention in writing this chapter to record the historical truth. It was to accept the likely truths behind my family's past as I understand them from family stories. Historical accounts of the period have allowed me to access the horror of those times in a way that I cannot connect with through my mother's oral history. Barnett's book on The Confessing Church, a movement within the German protestant community that arose in opposition to government-sponsored efforts to nazify the German Protestant Church, made for depressing reading and gave me no self-justifying narrative that could make my grandparents the exception to other Germans of their generation. Instead, it offered hellish complexity through the many first-hand accounts by confessing church members. My grandparents lived for their Christianity and had to face the task that lay ahead in rebuilding a church that had completely failed and was morally bankrupt. This reading lead me to a bleak place and allowed me to project a fresh mental image of my Opa, in the last years of his life as a sick, elderly man weighed down by the burden of it all.

Returning to the beginning – Black Lives Matter and anti-racism – I can see that 'White fragility' is real and the guilt and shame at its centre have parallels with other times and contexts. Social and cognitive psychologists see guilt as regret that an action has harmed another, thus it is rooted in empathy without the fear of retaliation that psychoanalytic readings lend it. In contrast, shame instils a sense of the self being irredeemably bad, deficient or defective. We all try to avoid experiencing shame by putting up a defence against accusations coming our way, real or perceived. In our attempt to sidestep the pain of shame, we lose our empathy for others while guilt is more likely to motivate us to reach out and make amends.

According to this definition we can see that *Vergangenheitsaufarbeitung*, German society's attempts to make amends for its past, is operating from a position of guilt rather than shame. By contrast 'white fragility' as defined by Diangelo can be seen as functioning from a place of shame that needs to be denied and dispelled at all costs. I hope that the process of *Vergangenheitsaufarbeitung* can be learned from and our collective commitment to creating a fairer, less racist society will be able to withstand the knocks and setbacks on the road ahead.

References

BACP. *Counselling skills competence framework (bacp.co.uk)*.

Barnett V. (1992) *For the soul of the people, protestant protest against Hitler*: New York, Oxford University Press.

Coles P. (2019) *The uninvited guest from the unremembered past. An exploration of the unconscious transmission of trauma across the generations*: London, Routledge.

Diangelo R. (2019) *White fragility: Why it's so hard for white people to talk about racism*: London, Allen Lane, Penguin Books.

Hammerich B., Pfafflin J. et al. in Gobodo Madikizela (2016) *Breaking intergenerational cycles of repetition: Global dialogue on historical trauma and memory;* Barbara Budrich Verlag (2016) Pumla Gobodo Madikizela: Chapter 13 'Handing down the holocaust in Germany: A reflection on the dialogue between second generation descendants of perpetrators and survivors' Beata Hammerich, Johannes Pfafflin, Peter Pogany-Wnendt, Erda Siebert, Bernd Sonntag.

Health & Care Professions Council HCPC 2013 *Standards of proficiency arts therapists* P8, 5.1–5.2 *(hcpc-uk.org)*.

Kahn M. (2020) Vox Highlight. The German model for America: The long and public reckoning that followed the Holocaust shows a path forward for a United States that desperately needs to confront its racist past. Updated Oct 5, 2020, 8:05am EDT. https://www.vox.com/the-highlight/21405900/germany-holocaust-atonement-america-slavery-reparations

Kaslow F. W. (2000 April) The fifth Holocaust dialogue interactive group session: Lessons to be learned *Journal of Marital and Family Therapy* Vol 26 No 2 pp 253–259.

Marcuse H. (2005 March) trans. The Stuttgart declaration of guilt. University of Santa Barbara https://marcuse.faculty.history.ucsb.edu/projects/niem/StuttgartDeclaration.htm.

Neiman S. (2020) *Learning from the Germans – Confronting race and the memory of evil*: London, Penguin Radom House.

Paulgaard J. The Confessing Church in Germany 1933 to 1945 *essay written for History 285.6, University of Saskatchewan, 8 April 1999 published February 9th 2009 at The Confessing Church in Germany 1933–45 – Farewell to Shadowlands (jamespaulgaard.com)*.

Payrhuber G. In the realm of the undead: Transgenerational transference and it's enactments *The British Journal of Psychotherapy Integration* Vol 8 No 1 pp 27–46.

Saad L. and DiAngelo R. (2020) *Me and white supremacy: How to recognise your privilege, combat racism and change the world*: London, Quercus.

Volkan V. (2002) *The Third Reich in the unconscious*: New York, Routledge.

Chapter 12

My story, our story

Co-parenting two adopted boys

Tony McLeod

My story starts in July 2014, the day my two adopted sons were placed with me and my partner Mark. I am black and British-born with Guyanese and Trinidadian roots, from a very traditional working-class family. Mark is white English, born in Kent and comes from a conventional English middle-class family. The boys reflect our mixed backgrounds. While they share the same birth mother, Alan is mixed heritage black Caribbean and white and Freddie is white. As their birth fathers were not available to them, Mark and I were to become the only fathers they have ever known. Eager as we were to co-parent, nothing prepared us for the, at times, heart-breakingly confusing and emotionally challenging experiences we were to face. I'm fortunate in having experience as a school-based behaviour specialist although I chose to stop work and become a full-time parent when we adopted Alan and Freddie. Yet the background skills and knowledge I possessed weren't sufficient to meet the needs of our children. As I describe in this still unfolding story, I had to be prepared to search out new ways of understanding and relating to the two very unique and now much-loved boys with whom Mark and I have had the privilege of co-creating our family. I imagine that my account of trauma-informed therapeutic parenting will be of interest to therapists and teachers who work with neurodiverse pupils or who are themselves parents of such children.

Alan was almost three years old when he was first removed from his mother Jane and then five when placed with us. Jane was reported to social services because Alan had acquired a number of unexplained marks on his body whilst in the care of Jane and her then partner, who was Freddie's birth father. This man was possibly the perpetrator of Alan's bruising and had been violent to Jane while she was pregnant. Consequently, Freddie too may have been exposed to trauma while in utero. Freddie was also removed from Jane's care at just four months old.

We were approved to adopt Alan and Freddie when they were five years old and 18 months old, respectively. Their journey to us involved a long battle of court proceedings. Their birth mother took on the local authorities in an attempt to retain parental responsibility. The courts ultimately agreed that the brothers would be safer in an adopted family but removing the boys from a

DOI: 10.4324/9781003270447-13

situation that was deemed unsafe took time. When it became clear that Jane was unable to protect her children, the boys were placed in two separate foster placements while the local authority processed the final adoption order.

It was a process that took a year, starting in 2012. By then the boys' trauma had already started to impact both of them, particularly Alan, and continues to do so. In the first instance, there was the impact of the issues that led to social services involvement in the first place. Additional trauma was experienced when the boys were taken away from their birth mother and put into foster care. Inevitably they were to experience further emotional upheaval when we came along. Finding a 'forever family' – a term used by some child welfare and adoption agencies, professionals, and families – is always a good thing, but moving from yet another home after leaving their original homes and then foster families can, for some children, result in re-traumatisation.

The cumulative effects of trauma and loss that my children have experienced in their short lives have resulted in their distrust and fear of adults. They firmly believe they can only depend on themselves as individuals, not even on each other. Despite our efforts to help them create a brotherly bond, each of them is bound up tightly in their trauma. When Mark and I came along, I feared that our sons were about to be traumatised again. From our perspective we were coming in to save the day, making their lives happier and more stable. But by setting up a new life together with us, they were being taken away, for the second time in their lives, from everything that was familiar to them after being in foster care for the best part of two years: a lifetime for children so young. Removing them from their foster carers would have a massive emotional impact on them and everyone around them, resulting in the internalisation of this event in their lives as yet another loss.

The pre-adoption process is intrusive but necessarily so in order to assess if the prospective adoptive parents have what it takes to care for traumatised children, and all that this inevitably involves. As part of that close examination, our social worker Claire challenged us to dig deep into our past to truly reflect on how we were raised and how we dealt with any trauma we may have experienced in our own lives. She left us drained, exposed, and vulnerable at times, but I can see why now. Being able to put our feet into our boys' shoes has been invaluable and enhances our powers of empathy with them, or at least our attempts at this. Both Mark and I have experienced trauma in our lives: rejection, alcoholism, grief, and loss as children and young people. Living through those challenges has made us who we are today. After much counselling as individuals and then coming together in adulthood, we have been able to process those experiences and make sense of them.

Our sons' experiences, like everyone's, have shaped their attachment styles. Alan enacted his avoidant orientation clearly and vividly from the very beginning. The first glimpse we had of it was when we walked into his foster family's house to bring him home with us: he ran and hid, only emerging after his foster mother coaxed him into coming out from behind the sofa. Freddie was – and remains – different. He was a toddler and came straight into our arms like it was the most natural thing to do. His foster carer and family cried more than he did the day we arrived to take him to our home. To this day he remains ambivalently attached. Despite the behaviours we saw in both boys, Mark and I remained upbeat that we could make a difference and create the family we had always dreamed of.

'Introductions' is the term given to the two weeks of preparatory meetings before children transition from foster care to their forever families. It's an intense period for everyone while adopters get to know the children and gain an understanding of how to care for them. The meetings are designed to minimise the risk of re-traumatising the children. It was, in fact, a grinding fortnight which left us feeling exhausted and emotional but, we felt, more prepared for the challenge of becoming Alan and Freddie's parents. While Freddie appeared to adjust relatively quickly to his new life with us, Alan began pushing back on the boundaries and routines we needed to lay down to keep him safe. Looking back, we were so naïve at the beginning. I thought my years of helping to care for my younger siblings alongside my professional experience and both our combined histories of looking after nieces and nephews would equip us with the skills and insights we needed to become the parents of traumatised children.

Our social worker advised us to start as we were to go on by setting clear rules and routines. However, with all the guidance in the world, nothing prepared us for the way the boys reacted to this, particularly Alan. He would have serious emotional outbursts or tantrums, not surprising considering his past and the defences he had developed in response to it, but nonetheless incredibly challenging to deal with. Over the following weeks and months Mark and I came to the conclusion that the children's behaviour needed to change. This was against the backdrop of Mark having returned to work, leaving me as the primary carer for the boys.

Realising that we would be needing help from social services, we had postponed applying for the adoption order that formalises the transition of parental responsibility from Jane to us and gives the boys our name. Our reason for the delay was so that social services would continue to have a duty of care to the children and to us, which we clearly needed and would lose when we became the boys' legal parents. It was, in other words, a safety net for getting help. Or so we thought. Instead, the message from social services was that we were doing well, that our expectations were too high, and that we needed to go on a parenting course. And so I duly signed up for one put on by the local authority's Early Help Team. I soon realised that I was something of a novelty as fathers, let alone a gay adoptive dad, rarely attended. While the course didn't give me the help I was looking for it brought me to the understanding that I would benefit from the support of a network to break through the isolation I was feeling.

This led me to Ann, a local adoptive mum who our social worker directed me to after a few months. She helped me reframe my children's behaviour and offered me support with my feelings of being alone in my new role. She got what I was going through and made me feel heard. I've lost count of the number of times she gave me space in her house to vent. Because Ann was active in the community, she soon introduced me to other mums, but still not many dads. Even so, our community grew until eventually we established We are Family (WAF), an adoption community.

Initially we started off as a group of parents with children of similar ages meeting up in the park for adult connection and play. After some time, we added a fortnightly support group that met without the children. I'm proud of my involvement with WAF, which has developed into a recognised charity as well as being the go-to community group for adopters and prospective adopters. In those early months and years WAF enabled me to feel less isolated, making connections with like-minded people. But I still needed to develop my skills in dealing with and managing my children's behaviour at home.

By now Freddie and I were attending local authority-run play groups where I met and engaged with professionals who I naively approached for support. In hindsight I can see that with no experience or training in trauma and or adoption they were not best placed to help. I was encouraged to join The Incredible Years Parenting Programme based on the Webster-Stratton model and delivered by a children's centre. I attended with an open mind but soon realised that the programme used a rewards and punishment model to manage children's behaviour which is dependent on the child being neurotypical and having an understanding of cause and effect. Research carried out by Adoption UK (2009) found that adopted parents who drew on standard programmes such as the Incredible Years model found that these models were inappropriate for children who have endured trauma and in fact could re-traumatise children because of the disciplinarian approach they are based on (as cited in Naish 2016). We found this out for ourselves over the next few years and increasingly I felt the need for something more concrete. My now well-established WAF network introduced me to Hand in Hand, Parenting by Connection (https://www.handinhandparenting.org) and The Great Behaviour Breakdown (Post, B 2009). Even though these paradigms were beginning to articulate more closely the kind of parent I wanted to be, they didn't quite fit. In the midst of those difficult times Mark and I moved house, bringing yet more change and upheaval into the lives of our transition-averse children. As we settled down in our new home, which was better suited to our needs, we began to explore the thinking behind something we'd heard about called 'therapeutic parenting' and attempted to start applying it.

My experience of therapeutic parenting

Therapeutic parenting, according to Sarah Naish of the National Association of Therapeutic Parenting (NATP), is the term used to describe an approach for parents who care for children with a history of trauma. I first stumbled on it when our social worker sent a round-robin email to adoptive parents offering a year's free subscription to NATP. Not knowing what I was getting into, I initially joined because it was free and it sounded like something that would help us. What soon became clear was that this was a parenting approach that not only reflects my own values and makes sense to our family and to us as parents but also gives me a sense of community that I have longed for since having children.

NATP founder Sarah Naish, who is UK based, began developing the therapeutic parenting model in 2007 in response to her research looking into the impact on parents of raising children with early life trauma. Through Sarah's work, I first came across the term developmental trauma to describe the attachment issues of children with a trauma-based background. Others in the field who support Sarah's work on trauma, such as psychotherapist Dan Hughes and Bruce Perry, a neuroscientist specialising in trauma, argue that the impact of neglect and abuse on child development can affect the growth of neural pathways. One of the consequences is attachment difficulties associated with developmental trauma. Sarah Naish argues that therapeutic parenting can help rewire those pathways in the brain when a child is able to make a strong connection with a consistent, boundaried, and nurturing parent. This rewiring can lead, among many other things, to the child's capacity to link cause and effect.

I have come to appreciate how therapeutic parenting also recognises the overwhelming feelings parents experience when trying to re-parent children with developmental trauma. Therapeutic parenting and NATP gave me access to peer support and resources to develop and sustain the consistent parental presence and connection my children need, enabled by the PACE parenting model, which can facilitate connectedness and empathy.

The PACE model, designed by Dan Hughes (as cited in Naish, 2018), provides a structure for my thinking and tools that encourage me to remain a responsive, loving, and boundaried parent.

PACE is an acronym for:

- Playfulness – A sense of humour helps create connection and allows de-escalation in moments of heightened emotion.
- Acceptance –Accepting our children for who they are and being prepared for them to make mistakes because of their challenging past
- Curiosity – Wondering aloud what needs or feelings they may be communicating.
- Empathy – Always responding with kindness and understanding by putting yourself in their shoes.

Parenting children from a trauma background is undeniably challenging. It can evoke intense feelings of isolation, failure, guilt, and shame in parents: all unhelpful reactions when the essence of what you are trying to do requires you to be fully present and emotionally responsive. Implicit in the concept of good enough therapeutic parenting is the understanding and acceptance that self-care is essential. While we all aim to be the best parent possible, Sarah Naish recognises that under extreme circumstances, it is difficult to remain so all the time: most of the time is good enough. A mantra that helps me overcome some of those feelings of guilt or shame and sometimes isolation when I have got it wrong is 'we are only human'. To help parents look after themselves, online therapeutic support groups offer the opportunity to meet like-minded people who understand and share similar challenges. The mutual empathy that is a cornerstone of these groups is an essential ingredient we need in order to function as a consistent and attuned parent and to help minimise many of the negative feelings that can so easily emerge.

I make it my self-care activity, particularly on those difficult days, to join a listening circle, which is a safe space for parents to get support from each other. They are non-judgmental groups run one or two hours a week by parent volunteers who are also therapeutic parents. Circle participants may signpost each other to strategies or agencies they have used, rather than offer solutions or advice.

While we need to be consistent in order to be good enough parents, there are times when we can be overwhelmed with the sense that there is no respite, leading to a state of blocked care or compassion fatigue. According to Sarah Naish (Naish, 2016 and 2018), compassion fatigue describes the feeling of emotional exhaustion; as a defence against this and to protect ourselves, we put some distance between ourselves and our children. The listening circle provides parents with the opportunity to 'fill up' on self-care, reduce the self-protection instinct in the brain, and bounce back into parenting. Given that our job as parents is to provide compassion for our children who may never have received it as well as to avoid overwhelming feelings of fatigue in ourselves, self-care is as important for our children as for their parents.

Boundaries and routines

For the nine years that we have been a family I have been the primary carer for Alan and Freddie. I stopped working soon after they arrived because the impact of their disturbing histories on their young lives soon became apparent, and my returning to work ran the risk of exacerbating their mental health even further. My parenting strategy at the time was to follow the only model I had at that point: the way I was parented. I grew up in a traditional West Indian home where strict boundaries and routines dominated. This was the only model I knew and both Mark and I realised we were getting it wrong in those early days. However, the boundaries and routines we introduced from the beginning have remained foundational for us as a family as well as being fundamental to the therapeutic parenting approach.

One such boundary is that the boys are not allowed to have any technology in their bedrooms overnight. They know that this is to avoid the risk of them staying up all night. Still, there have been occasions when a device has ended up in Alan's bedroom after lights out. On one occasion the natural consequence was that Alan was so exhausted the following morning that he could not join in on a family excursion. Not being able to get up that day, he saw for himself that the result of choosing to stay up playing games was that he couldn't participate in a fun activity: a vivid example not of punishment but of cause and effect.

Keeping to the rules avoids direct intervention from the parents; instead it gives us the opportunity to use empathy and to explain cause and effect. It is through examples like this that the PACE model of therapeutic parenting provides a strong conceptual and practical framework. It allows me to step back and reflect on what is going on. I may not use playfulness on such occasions but I do accept that the boys are unable to control themselves at times. I can empathise with them when they get it wrong while at the same time, lovingly insisting that the boundary in our house remains: no technology in the bedroom.

Our approach to routines is illustrated in how we approach bedtimes. In our home Alan and Fred go to bed at the same time every night, regardless of whether it's a school night, weekend or holiday. My children spend a lot of time in what I call 'toddler brain' because of their troubled early experiences and consequent disorganised attachment pattern. The impact of developmental trauma is that sometimes they can get stuck or switch between their cognitive and their chronological ages, moving between reactive, irrational and/or recalcitrant toddler behaviour to being the 14- and ten-year-olds they are at other times. What it means for a therapeutic parent is that having this idea in my mind helps me to have realistic expectations of them, giving me the capacity to reflect, understand and manage the situation with empathy and firmness.

So, a good enough therapeutic parent responds to cognitive age at any given time and, in the example above, sets a bedtime routine that meets the child's needs. We have learned our lesson when the children stay up late: the next day, they can be tired and become dysregulated and hard to manage for everyone. It is better to be realistic about what our children can handle. An early night or two for parents is also essential for our well-being.

How to manage dysregulation as a therapeutic parent

Dysregulation and regulation are common words in our house and in the world of therapeutic parenting. What we call 'wobbly' is another one, referring to the overwhelming urge they can have, for instance, to crawl around on the floor like a toddler. Psychiatrist Bruce Perry describes how the neurons become hardwired or fixed following an experience such as neglect. When that hardwiring leads Alan to distrust all adults, the amygdala, the part of the brain that processes fearful and threatening signals and is in charge of responses to threat and danger, fires warnings. This occurs particularly at times of transitions, which may be experienced as existential threats. Alan can become very wobbly and dysregulated when perceiving a threat which triggers instinctual fight, flight or freeze modes. My awareness of the fact that he can't help these responses helps keep me grounded. I accept this and can reflect with curiosity on his early life and the causes for these reactions.

These behaviours can be unlearned: the experience of being therapeutically parented encourages the child's brain to relax and ultimately counter the hyper-vigilance to threat in the absence of external threat. This takes time. Speaking to different adoptive parents, I have heard various views on the timescale that rewiring can take. Some say eight or ten years, others not until children are into adulthood. My children have been with me for nine years now and we are still dealing with fight, flight, and freeze responses, necessitating our need to repeatedly demonstrate to them in different ways that they are safe.

A therapeutic approach to transitions

Gillian Schofield and Mary Beek of BAAF Adoption and Fostering recommend that parenting strategies must be sensitive and considered to support the child through difficult transitions. In the world of fostering and adoption unfortu-nately there can be many transitions: children can be moved around the care system multiple times, with every move risking the possibility of regression. Child psychology shows us time and again the primacy of consistency and se-curity in the growth of children's sense of well-being (Li, 2022). But in the care system, for a variety of reasons, some of which are unavoidable, the lack of consistency can result in serious distress.

If not handled sensitively, these transitions can trigger an instant reaction that can impact its successful outcome. This includes both big changes such as moving school or home to smaller ones like going on holiday – basically any deviation from the accustomed routine. In our house, we try to carefully manage transitions drawing on several strategies to support the boys during these times. The key to this is accepting that the boys will find change difficult no matter how much we plan. Therefore, we will often delay telling them about something different which is about to happen and that might cause anticipa-tory anxiety. For example, joining a new holiday camp they have never been to can provoke a reaction so we only share such vacation plans nearer the time, allowing minimum scope for anxiety. Another strategy is to work alongside them to help them stay regulated. I will often co-regulate transitioning which means staying side by side with them to model the behaviour I would like them to adopt or to distract them while they navigate the transition.

As might have become clear in my description so far, therapeutic parenting can sometimes be tedious as it involves a lot of repetition. For instance, to min-imise transition anxiety we regularly revisit the same holiday places. While not our first choice or at all adventurous, I've come to appreciate going back to the same cottage in the country or family-friendly hotel in Spain because familiarity minimises the boys' anxieties. They feel safe in a place they've been before with less chance of surprises, threats, or something unexpected happening. They're more likely to be happy and relaxed and because they are, we are.

Therapeutic parenting and schools

Schooling is a major pillar in all children's lives. For many parents, the worry of how to get theirs into the best schools begins to preoccupy them from the earliest years. For parents like me with emotionally challenged children, the battle is not for high academic standards as much as to find a trauma-informed school. According to Louise Bomber (2007), a teacher and therapist, this is the kind of school which recognises that students may have been exposed to trauma or loss and, as a result, may demonstrate behavioural and cognitive challenges.

Louise Bomber says that to meet these children in education, schools need to adapt and become more inclusive. A trauma-aware school mirrors the approach I attempt to follow at home: adjusting my responses to the children's needs as much as possible and recognising that their behaviour tends to be the result of their troubled past. Therefore, when the behaviour is not acceptable, I try to help the boys experience the natural consequences of that behaviour. When they are ready to hear, I provide an explanation, simple messages and repetition of those messages and, in extreme cases, I will temporarily remove items like phones to support the messages. At home we try to use a nurturing response to address difficult behaviours alongside empathy and curiosity. I am fortunate to have children who respond to this approach, but we are far from the finished product.

It goes without saying that in most school settings there is little or no room for a more considered approach to disruptive behaviour. The expectation is that irrespective of their particular backgrounds, pupils will conform to the rules. When this doesn't happen, sanctions such as detentions and exclusions are applied with parents being called in for meetings. All of this can be felt as a form of punishment rather than more considered attempts to address the needs of troubled children. I have had the painful experience of Alan suffering the consequences of his school's rigid rules. I used to dread the school pick-up where the teacher was often at the class door, catching my eye and indicating he needed a word as Alan had hit someone or refused to do something, which the teacher described as 'being naughty'. It was a frustrating time as school policies dictated that this is how the teacher should respond to challenging behaviour. That Alan had moved home just months previously and had started at a new school was not taken into account by the staff. But what I knew was that when Alan acted out at school his 'fear brain' had been activated: his behaviour was an enactment of feeling unsafe. A more therapeutic, trauma-informed response on the part of the teacher would have been to look behind the behaviour in an attempt to understand it and to respond with more empathy and compassion. However, I am fully aware of how difficult a task this can be when dealing with a number of similarly challenging behaviours in a class of 25–30. This is especially so as mainstream teachers and classroom assistants are rarely offered training in trauma-sensitive teaching and disciplinary strategies.

Adoptive parents spend a lot of time and energy searching for that perfect school which can demonstrate trauma and attachment-informed behaviour policies. I believe that such a school should be able to apply behaviour policies that reflect their understanding of the impact of trauma on children's behaviour and the challenges those children face in following school rules. Those specialist teachers who have this awareness have the potential to inform and influence behaviour policy. The reality, of course, can be very different. My heart sinks when a supposedly specialist teacher compares neurotypical children's behaviour with my developmentally traumatised child's behaviour to show she understands. This is unhelpful and serves to drive home the point that such teachers would benefit not only from regular refresher courses but also supervision to provide containment and thinking space. I know what it is like to try to parent without ongoing support so I can imagine what teachers might go through.

My therapeutic practice as a parent has had a constructive influence on my professional work within the limits of school policy. For example, as a behaviour specialist I draw on the PACE approach to behaviour management. This means that when dealing with challenging behaviour, I have the tools to de-escalate situations without reverting to punitive actions. I have found that adopting a nurturing, empathic tone has helped me deflate emotionally heightened situations.

In my time in education, I have seen both students and teachers become dysregulated as they compete to be heard. I'm aware, as a staff member and as a parent, of the responsibility we have to children to role-model the behaviour we want them to adopt. The same could be said about our interactions with parents. As school staff, we don't know the baggage parents carry from their own school experiences, informing their engagement with staff as representatives of the school. Given the possibility that their schooling was problematic, the PACE model can be useful in facilitating parents' meetings, drawing on acceptance of possible negativity and showing empathy.

A blog from an adoptive parent once commented that you never really know if a school is trauma-informed until you get there. For parents of adopted children it is particularly important to develop a relationship with the school in order to best support them. I spend a lot of time speaking to Alan's school about interventions and strategies. Transitions within education are difficult at the best of times for most families practicing therapeutic parenting but my experience of working in partnership can help bridge the gap between home and school with the aim of providing a team around the child with a common goal.

Conclusion

Therapeutic parenting is challenging, exhausting and sometimes counter intuitive. But it is necessary when parenting children with developmental trauma. Everyday life with children like Alan and Freddie can feel extreme and even at times a matter of life or death. We know that early experiences are embedded in the brain, leading to sometimes difficult attachment patterns. To manage this, therapeutic parenting offers a nurturing and empathic base to help regulate those warning signals in the brain, over-riding feelings of threat and distrust. Through clear boundaries and established routines, I have begun to address those fears in my children, but it is a long process which may not yield behaviour change for years to come. As part of this approach, Dan Hughe's PACE model is a powerful framework that helps me manage their dysregulation and the inevitable transitions they face in their lives. It also allows me space to reflect on what is going on in the midst of difficult moments. While changes that are part and parcel of ordinary life may always be difficult for children with troubled histories, the PACE model gives therapeutic parents a structure to minimise the effects of trauma that may rear their head at any time.

Therapeutic parenting involves an understanding of your child's needs, where those needs come from and strategies to help them overcome the everyday challenges they face. Dealing with schools, where priorities are not necessarily in synch with your own, is one of the biggest challenges. Typically, the majority of schools still use a punishment and reward approach to managing behaviour with the inherent risk of reinforcing the unspoken message that the child is not good enough or worthy. Cause and effect, which is the foundation of reward and punishment models, does little to change behaviour in children such as mine. When they get it wrong, a hug and an empathic reaction get a more positive response from them than punitive action. As an educationalist I have also seen first-hand the consequences of the same children repeatedly falling foul of rules and policies. Since it is not possible to know how behaviour is dealt with in practice until your child experiences the reward and sanction system first-hand, the best approach parents can adopt is attempting to work in partnership with schools. While a hug and empathy aren't realistic expectations of pressurised school staff, a heightened awareness of the story behind a child's behaviour may elicit more considered and empathic responses when trouble arises.

Therapeutic parenting has become a central part of our lives, giving me, as the primary carer in our family, a structure to work within when meeting head-on some of the difficulties that arise with our children. An essential component to this approach, given the isolation, guesswork and sometimes frustrations of parenting troubled children, is self-care. Failing to look after ourselves invites the risk of tipping into compassion fatigue or blocked care, resulting in disconnecting and losing the capacity to support the children.

For the next stage of my journey as a therapeutic parent with the attendant need to look after myself, I will return to work and will be seeking therapeutic childcare – a tall order and probably hard to find. As for the boys, I have hopes and dreams that they will become better adjusted to who they are, that they will learn to trust, love and find happiness. But we also know they will always have a trauma-based background and therefore need and deserve a model of age-appropriate therapeutic support throughout their lives.

References

Bomber, L.M. (2007) *Inside I'm Hurting.* London: Worth Publishing Ltd.

Hand in Hand: https://www.handinhandparenting.org/.

Li, P. (2022) *Bowlby and Ainsworth Attachment Theory – How Does It Work.* On parentingforbrain.com/attachment-theory.

Naish, S. (2016) *Therapeutic Parenting in a Nutshell: Positives and Pitfalls.* London: Jessica Kingsley.

Naish, S. (2018) *The A-Z of Therapeutic Parenting: Strategies and Solutions.* London: Jessica Kingsley.

National Association of Therapeutic Parenting: https://www.naotp.com/.

Post, B. (2009) *The Great Behaviour Breakdown.* Palmyra VA: Post Institutes and Associates.

Schofield, G. and Beek, M. (2006) *Attachment Handbook for Foster Care and Adoption.* London: British Association for Adoption and Fostering.

We are Family Adoption: https://wearefamilyadoption.org.uk/.

Chapter 13

One of many

The impact of growing up in a large family

Margery Craig

> *All my family had too many children, including my parents. None of them know when to stop.*
>
> *Eva, aged 14*

One outcome of a psychotherapeutic training is that we tend to internalise the template of an ideal therapist, the one we 'should' be. But the person we really are in the room is far from a pattern book clone. What we attune to, what we hear acutely, and what we always miss or resist exploring and even our resistance to the transference itself, will reveal aspects of who we are despite our best efforts. Resistance is not one-sided. Our client may defend against intrusion, but we too resist understanding the unprocessed parts of ourselves that we do not want to meet again. However, in most cases, our resistance does not derail the therapy and with enough adherence to our method, coupled with our client's hope that we will be helpful, we are able to build a good enough therapeutic relationship to be of use.

Young people do not always come with a desire for help or a 'cure', especially not when we are working with the hyper-vigilant adolescent. They may have organised their defences around a very fragile and loosely constructed self, mobilised to protect against question, criticism, or ridicule, avoiding or staving off every attempt to make contact. In these circumstances we may be subtly or overtly mocked or simply ignored if we stay in the relative neutrality of the therapist's role. But if we are provoked into a more active stance or get caught up in our own relationship with what is at stake, we risk saying more about ourselves than we do about them, obliterating what small clues there are in front of us, thereby confirming the young person's basic assumption that no one can be of any use to them.

The developmental processes of adolescence, always in dynamic relationship with whatever family exists, can be extremely painful and involve the risk of destabilisation. Young people we meet are in the throes of separation from a state in which they have until now been 'described' by others and are beginning the process of defining themselves. It is no wonder that symptoms designed

DOI: 10.4324/9781003270447-14

to hold the self together emerge during this process. And this is where the personal comes into the picture, as I reflect not just on others but also on how I experienced myself described as 'one of many', perhaps one of too many demanding siblings, and how I built a defensive structure to avoid the very unsettling yet mundane truth of this.

Beginnings

As I would with a client, I've chosen to explore my family of origin as a starting point, a family that was at times over-stretched and emotionally under-resourced in a way that was both particular, and yet not untypical, of its time and place. I will be thinking more broadly about the implications of this for a child's developing self, including the often-deleterious effects of the unconscious assumption that there is 'not enough to go around'. However, I will also be asking to what extent a sense of 'lack' can be seen as a creation of the child's mind rather than a defining feature of their environment. I want to stress that this is not a critique of large families; a child with many siblings can flourish, feeling securely held in mind; and conversely an 'only' child might experience a deficiency in their parents' emotional availability or attunement. Nor will the theme of 'one of many' be placing the emphasis on a shortage of love. A parent can love their children but may struggle with emotional unavailability or with feelings of ambivalence because they themselves are under-resourced materially or emotionally or have not had sufficiently good experiences of being parented themselves. There are as many histories as there are individuals in a family and what we construct is rarely an accurate representation of what has gone on in our formative years. We know as therapists that constructions can be fluid, and we will most likely arrive at new constructions if we continue to till the intrapsychic soil.

I will be attempting to set out a small part of my family story as factually as I can, whilst acknowledging that facts have limited value in the analytic economy. What has formed us is not what is 'true' but what we have come to believe, often based on what we have been told in our family, including the snippets we have gleaned from what was not meant for us to hear, all of which become our conscious 'knowns'. This is what is synthesised into the subject we become, and what organises the narrative we construct about ourselves and others. Much unwanted and unprocessed material will have been relegated to the unconscious, alive yet unincorporated: the 'unconscious knowns'. I am also aware that the way I tell my story, and what I include or leave out, emphasise or downplay, is specific to me, and that each person in my family will have a different take on it, none being 'wrong' and none holding all the truth.

Family context

My parents could be described as being on the cusp of the so-called 'Silent Generation', a term used to define those who came of age during the Second

World War. In 1939, as the war was declared, my mother was 12, the eldest of three children, with a younger sister and brother. Although she remained in her home city of Glasgow throughout the war, it could have been a very different story. The threat in Europe was such that my grandparents had signed up for their children to be evacuated to Canada as part of the Children's Overseas Reception Board, a British government-sponsored organisation. My mother would have been preparing herself for a caretaking role for her siblings. That plan was abandoned when the evacuee ship assigned to this task was torpedoed on an Atlantic crossing, killing 77 children on board. So their lives in Glasgow continued. In support of the war effort and in keeping with 'the auld alliance', my grandparents accepted the billeting of Free French soldiers in their home, something perhaps both exciting and disturbing for them and their children.

My father was 14 at the start of the war, the eldest of two with a younger sister. When his parents moved from Glasgow to Belfast to maintain my grandfather's job as a crane engineer in the shipyards, my father remained in Glasgow with his mother's unmarried sisters. At 18 he was conscripted and trained up for the D-Day landings, but instead served on a minesweeper, protecting merchant convoys. Surviving these supply passages must have been a cold, relentless numbers game from which my father returned in poor health. His father's aunt told us how he was given stout in hospital to build him up. We were amused at the idea of prescription alcohol but war-induced damage was often minimised, even denied. Nor was the link made in those days between the daily use of navy ration cigarettes and 'tots' of rum or gin to 'boost spirits' and the continuation of these forms of self-medication, and potentially addiction, in civilian life.

My mother went on to university to study French and German as her mother had done before her. The latter part of her course included a period of living and studying in post-war Paris. She came back strangely transformed, slim and soigné, with a French 'fiancé' who came to meet my grandparents and was hastily dispatched by them as unsuitable. I cannot help but wonder about the place of her own desire.

My father restored his own liveliness at university after the war and became involved in student politics and some high jinx, taking up a central role as both Liberal and Nationalist. It was at university my parents met through mutual friends and married. My father's mother had high hopes for her son's political ambition while my maternal grandmother may have had some ambivalence about my mother's fledgling role as a trainee fashion buyer, the sort of ambition my grandmother might well have had to put aside for herself, when in late adolescence, she and her siblings lost their parents and had to take on adult responsibilities. One of those siblings had a disability, that my grandmother, speaking to my aunt, referred to as 'not quite right', but in a tone of great affront, the indignancy that covers shame. My grandmother's need to keep up appearances led her to manage her own family with a critical eye and this way of being in the world was, I think, internalised in turn by my mother.

The post-war generation

My parents' generation was shouldering the financial debt of the country as well as the debt the living owed to those who had lost their lives in the war. It is hard to know how much this responsibility was felt by individuals, and how swiftly it would be forgotten. However, those beginning their careers at the time were expected to restore the economy and not least, to rebuild the population.

At the start of their married life, my parents moved to London, perhaps to escape their parents' desire, perhaps to fulfil it. My father had secured a job assisting the director of what became the CBI – the Confederation of British Industry. If my mother sacrificed her own career in Glasgow for his professional opportunities, it remained unstated.

My siblings and I knew little about their life before ours began, but we did know it was in London that they lost their first baby. I'm not sure how we gleaned an awareness of this despite both wanting and not wanting to know. My mother had few words with which to describe it and when asked, repeated it not as a story, but in a fragmentary way, speaking of a full-term birth with the midwives bundling away the baby boy she did not see, and being told he had been 'unviable'. Through the unprocessed horror colouring her account, we must have registered her fantasy, full of self-reproach, of having borne something 'monstrous', and maybe not 'still' at all. After this personal tragedy, my parents returned to Scotland via Yorkshire where my brother was born just a year later and then, in short order, my sister, myself and my younger brother, bringing the tally to four living children, still all under six years of age.

My father had relinquished political ambition and taken a job in manufacturing that involved long overseas trips. This left my mother parenting alone, usually for weeks at a time in a small town where she had no connections. It is hard not to speculate whether this was a way of my father making an escape from parenthood. Did he re-find himself in some of those exotic places, I wonder? As for my mother, why had she chosen a man who found it so painful to 'come down to earth', who would repeatedly leave her in charge? Was it an acceptance, like Wendy in J.M. Barrie's Peter Pan (2006) that she was destined to be the grown-up, or did she have difficulty in sharing her children with our father, a burden and a consolation that was to be hers alone?

Regardless, she needed help to be a mother and found it in Sir Frederic Truby King (1923), a New Zealand social worker, health reformer and Director of Child Welfare who promoted ideas such as 'feeding by the clock', that is, at precisely six hourly intervals and that babies should not be kept close to their mother: 'the pram in the garden' was to ensure distance and healthy fresh air. My mother followed this advice, the same child-rearing guidance her own mother would have used. King's baby care method, with its roots in patriotism, continued in popularity following two world wars and seemed predicated on a fear of the twin perils of a 'manipulative' infant and a mother's unhealthy entanglement with it. Perhaps fortunately, although too late for us, this was re-placed with the re-publication of 'The Common Sense Book of Baby and Child Care' by Benjamin Spock (1957) building on his revolutionary advice to moth-ers that 'you know more than you think you do – just follow your instincts'.

Expert advice is a comfort for many new parents and the guidance itself seems to matter less than whether the parents feel contained by their belief in the writer. My mother's adherence to King's severe strictures might be under-stood as an attempt to be the perfect maternal figure or at least to be beyond reproach, driven by the desire to refute the internalised critical mother, and of course, as an unconscious protection against another infant death. My aunt told me about visiting my mother in Yorkshire after my eldest brother was born and seeing her clear distress at my brother's remorseless howling in the other room whilst she stuck doggedly to King's orders to 'build character' by avoid-ing cuddling and attentiveness in general. At the time my aunt, herself still an adolescent, was aghast at her sister's loss of 'common sense'. I don't doubt that as more babies arrived, my mother did start to let go of the rulebook somewhat.

I don't remember my mother turning to her mother for help, yet I imagine it was hard for my grandmother to witness my mother's struggles. My memory of one of our few visits to my grandmother, who died when I was seven, was of her strict manner and her criticism of us four demanding children. Her be-haviour might be understood now, but not then, as an attempt to protect my mother from the relentlessness of her small children's needs. At the time we felt reproached, disliked, and altogether 'too much'. Meanwhile we enjoyed my grandfather's company hugely. The first person I heard described as 'eccentric', he was erudite but a hopelessly impractical *Puer aeternus* ('eternal boy') in the eyes of his wife and daughters, and thus delightfully willing and able to give himself over to play with his grandchildren.

Family life I

It is far from rare in therapy to hear from a client that their parents' marriage was unhappy, and they only stayed together 'for us'. But how can we really know about our parents' choices and the quality of their attachment to each other? Wrapped up in our own oedipal drives and the narcissistic pursuit of growing up, children can be biased and unreliable witnesses. Equally it would be impossible to try to quantify some sort of deficit of love in a dynamic family system based on what can be observed from the outside. A child's love of its parent can be a complicated, demanding, submissive, or rejecting love, just as a parent's love for a child can be ambivalent, underscored by unconscious desire, fear, envy, and aggression. Each demand will solicit or fail to solicit something from the other.

Nevertheless, in my mind there was an aura of depression and disappointment in our house as we grew up. When writing this, I was listening to Bernadine Evaristo's 'Manifesto' (2019). Hearing her describe her family of origin I had to question what makes one family a large rumbunctious banister-sliding playground of opportunity, and another a grey empty place. We too had a banister, over which I threw my sister's favourite doll. Was it envy that dampened the possibility of fun? It put me in mind of finding '*The Darling Buds of May*' (1958) on my parent's bookshelf when I was around 12 years old. I loved that family, bursting with familial pride and tolerance, and so did my parents apparently – so why could *we* not be like that?

* * * *

Birth order is steeped in meaning for parents based on their past experiences of their own siblings and their place in their own family. Prophecy Coles (2003) notes how little attention Freud paid to sibling relationships yet a child's developing self might well be overwritten by a family narrative about an uncle or aunt whose qualities are attributed to the child. My mother was a dutiful and academic older sister, like my older sister, while I was the younger one, of whom little but frivolity was expected, like my aunt. My eldest brother, the second to arrive but the first to survive, inevitably suffered from an excess of concern that he should be 'quite right'. By subsequently finding it difficult to fit in socially, he fulfilled the worrying destiny of being '*not* quite right'.

As therapists, when we speak to a young person, it is useful to find out who they think they are for their parents, and what meaning they give to their place in the family. It is likely that the sibling relationships in an emotionally under-resourced family take on a special importance, even a deadly one. Perhaps as Coles says, there is a tendency in us all to wish that we could be the only child, never having to compete for attention, ensuring that we are the most loved one. What do we do with this impossible wish? Do we long to obliterate our siblings, violently or by stealth, do we make them look bad so we can look good, or do we give up the competition and leave them to it, perhaps only to pick up hope again later in life? How many less favoured children have taken up the role of caring for a parent in later life in order to get the closeness that was previously devoted to a sibling? Some families try to reduce envy by being painstakingly fair, at the expense of individualism. Some children form caring alliances with a younger or older sibling to get their needs met that way or develop a symptom that gives them importance and which demands their parents' (or caring substitutes') attention. How do these ways of being in the world continue through our life?

The complexity of a sibling relationship is acutely observed in Phoebe Waller-Bridge's television series *Fleabag* (2016) in which the mother has died and the father is emotionally blocked. Though 'Fleabag' and her sister share the same loss and wish for their parents' love, their relationship has been marred by competition and wilful misunderstanding. This makes the tentative and imperfect rapprochement late in the series particularly joyful.

* * * *

During my therapy training I came across something that had a profound resonance for me. We were watching a 1969 documentary film by social workers
John and Joyce Robertson entitled 'John' about a child adapting to a residential
nursery setting. I saw an uncanny resemblance to my mother in the figure of
the lone depleted nursery worker sitting on the floor swamped by children, now
including John, all jostling for a place on her lap. Later in the film, we see John
progressively giving up on trying to find a meaningful connection and then a
final image that shocked me into emitting an involuntary loud convulsive sob,
of John listless and resigned, soothing himself with blanket and thumb.

I have no doubt that these films continue to be such a valuable but disquieting resource because made at a time when ethical considerations were very
different from today, they have captured part of a universal experience, blankets
and thumbs being classic substitutions for the absence of mother. And I wonder
whether my involuntary reaction was not only that I was seeing myself, who
remained attached to my blanket and thumb long after the norm, but also my
older brother, who was more remote than the rest of us, the proverbial 'lone wolf
howling in the wilderness'.

* * * *

As an infant starts to make sense of itself as a separate being, it relies on the
attunement of its first carer – most often the mother. Winnicott (1967) tells
us that early attunement and mirroring – that is, experiencing oneself as
being met and understood – is the catalyst for the formation of a cohesive self,
of being a subject rather than an inchoate bundle of scattered affects. Lacan
(1949) saw this mirror phase somewhat differently, ascribing to it the effect of
providing us with an *image* which, though it is not and never can be 'our self',
serves well enough as this. Our subjectivity seems to be captured in our image,
although we remain forever split between 'self' and 'image'. In health, perhaps
these are not so unrecognisably far apart.

On becoming a subject, a *someone*, we can start to take up our own agency,
and where parental care is stretched, for example with the birth of a sibling, we find our way to other substitutes for love and attention. This can be
developmentally ordinary and healthy, from adopting a transitional object to
seeking a top-up of attention from a favourite grandparent or carer. As we grow,
the outside world and the move towards autonomy entice us; school, sport, or
social activities, friendships, siblings, or animals might all provide compensatory
relationships, helping to soften the process of separation from mother. If there
is insufficient capacity for attunement or recognition or if there is a consistent
mis-recognition between the parent and infant, or an excess of ambivalence and
primitive anxieties, this fundamental process may fail.

What might have been enough for one infant may be insufficient for another,
and some children will approach the oedipal stage quite unprepared to navigate the numerous 'castrations' it entails. They might experience separation as

premature, a persecuting deprivation akin to starvation which they struggle to assuage. They may, within the limited resources of a child, develop strategies to recreate what has been lost. For example, some offer the care to others that they long for themselves, a tactic often misread and rewarded by adult approval. Others might employ a denial of their needs as their defence, coldly rejecting love or attention, or refusing food in an outward display of independence whilst finding secondary gratification elsewhere. These defensive solutions may be revisited in adolescence, the second stage of normal separation. However, riskier strategies for denying needs and asserting independence outside of the home draw some young people into behaviours that can potentially lead to unwanted or destructive coping strategies such as addiction to porn, substances misuse, or gambling.

It would be unhelpful and inaccurate to lay blame here either at the door of an over-stretched parent or an emotionally hungry child. If psychoanalytic thinking teaches us anything, it is that we are rarely simply victims of events. We must examine the part our own primitive aggression plays and our mastery, or not, of it. What we tell ourselves (and what our clients tell us) is rarely the whole story.

Family life 2

When I was a child, my maternal grandparents brought back a large, illustrated book from a trip to France for my sister and me to share. It was full of illustrations of elegant, costumed women. Inside the front cover was a pocket and inside this nestled a perfect miniature replica of the book exactly the same in every detail, only scaled down. Despite this being a charming assemblage, it brought up for me a deeply unsettling association: was I only a 'subset' of my sister, and what did this tell me about who she and I were for my grandparents? For years, keeping those two books together was fraught. My sister would open the large one and become anxious when the small one was missing, searching for it to return it to its rightful place. I meanwhile wanted to keep them apart, one each, equal and unconnected.

When I was small, I played in the street with neighbouring children, and as we got older, we ventured further afield, out of sight and sound of any adult. I thought of myself as the one in my family who was outward facing – 'street wise' – as I took part in these expeditions which my siblings did not. I was finding a solution to my problem of 'being', proving I was not one of a needy many, but different and independent. Perhaps too there was an unconscious desire to be missed. This pattern continued into adolescence. I had progressively given up trying to please in a very academic school where I was outclassed by my sister: I couldn't win so I didn't compete and by 16, fell for a man who was a good many years older. This relationship kept me out of the house once again but the strategy failed me when the relationship ended after two years. Though amicable, it was as if I was returned home and now 'un-illuminated' by this alternative love, I was confronted with my home's bleakness. My parents were wrapped in their own separate disappointments, near breaking point, and my older brother moved from room to room in the house as Françoise Dolto (1984) puts so well "like a spaceship without an astronaut". By now, my other two siblings had made a break for it, both attending university in a different city. I developed a symptomology – anorexia – perhaps to reassert that I needed no part of this 'affronting' household. Anorexia nervosa can be seen to function as an unconscious solution to psychological distress. Like other symptoms, it can best be understood by its specificity to the individual – that is, how *this* self and *this* body have arrived at *this* as a solution to a problem.

I had been a picky eater as far back as I could remember. It wasn't made a big deal of at home; my mother accommodated the exceptions each of us made for her food (and by association, for her). Remembering further back than I could, she told me it wasn't always thus and as an infant, I had an insatiable appetite for milk. At that time, I interpreted her words as criticism and strongly refuted this perception, thinking she had confused me with one of the others. After all, I knew I hated the school milk. Nevertheless, family photos do show me as a well filled out baby. Only later pictures taken around the time I was school age show me as the familiar small and slight child my older brother nicknamed 'skinny', a definition that distinguished me from the others. I wonder what passed between my mother and myself when I came to be weaned off my beloved milk? Was it simply my younger brother's arrival inevitably setting the limit? Or was there an intrapsychic choice to refute my need or greed?

How does anorexia nervosa start? Although my mother and older sister occasionally embarked on diets, this was their shared preoccupation. My position as 'the skinny one' meant I was unaffected by these concerns. However, in the summer when I turned 19, I had a holiday job in a remote Highland restaurant with friends where our post-shift social life revolved around food and drink and lots of it. A male friend, (perhaps standing-in as the arbiter of body size for my older brother) visited us late in the summer and noticed my too-tight jeans, remarking that I was no longer skinny. My reaction was instant. I stopped eating to rectify the irrefutable evidence of my greed and to reclaim my 'signifier'.

I shed that weight, but afraid of slipping back I continued to restrict what I ate. Back at college I was doing well and this may have played a part in my intrapsychic economy; perhaps ambition (greed?) had to be countered with literal self-diminishment, a sort of moral offsetting. But I was becoming quite unwell, physically fragile and disconnected from the real body others saw yet I could not truly see in my mirror. My family colluded, as we did over other things, blind to the symptoms. My friends too were silenced by my refusal to have this spoken about or to countenance any need of help.

Eventually, brought to a halt by an infection I could not shake, and after an uncharacteristic expression of concern by my older brother breaking through the silence, I declared an uneasy truce, allowing just enough recovery to get to the finishing line in college. I had worked doggedly and did achieve success but

I was still caught up in this symptom, when, about to turn 21, I left Glasgow for London with my portfolio and no plan beyond getting out. Like pulling off a plaster, it was a radical separation from home and all it stood for and perhaps represented an urgent attempt at self-cure.

Moving to a place where you know no one is a big deal as well as an opportunity for renewal. Arriving on my own and unprepared in London, I had to become robust enough to stand on my own. This was not a conscious process, and for a long time I simply rode the tide of events, surviving, observing, free-floating. Consciously, I busied myself addressing the most basic of the hierarchy of needs first – food, shelter, and work. Gradually, friendships and new identifications were formed as, over the years, I carved out a new life for myself, making London my permanent 'home from home', the city where I still live today.

Clinical resonance

Adolescence and young adulthood is a time when loosening attachment bonds and trying out new identifications becomes necessary. Without a solid base, this process can be particularly precarious and it is not uncommon in these cases for a young person to develop early coping mechanisms which become increasingly problematic in adolescence. So it was with Eva, a young person I saw in a large secondary school early in my counselling career.

The school had referred her, concerned about what lay behind Eva's failure to engage academically or in the wider life of the school. There was an air of neglect as if no parental mind contained her. The school had told me about the family's situation and stretched resources, and that although her parents had attended meetings they had called about Eva, school staff felt frustrated by what they experienced as her parents' passivity and apparent powerlessness to even think about Eva's difficulties. Her parents had been barely adults them-selves when they had their first child; perhaps their superficial compliance with the school may have masked anger at the inherent power imbalance in their situation. With what they experienced as a seemingly unbridgeable chasm of class and culture between them and the teachers, Eva's parents reacted to any attempt at understanding their circumstances as implied criticism.

When I met Eva, she insisted all was 'fine' with her, emphasising that the school's concerns were trivial and that she was perfectly able to look after herself without help. She thought it 'ridiculous' that the school and I, by association, were questioning this. When asked about her family, she said there was nothing to say, then threw out the insight that everyone in the whole of her extensive network of relations had too many children, her parents included. She added that none of them knew when to stop, her parents having had 'at least one too many'.

Whilst I acknowledged the words, I did not open up the conversation, making a judgement in the moment that it was too soon to unpack such potent material, containing what I took to be a scarcely veiled allusion to murderous fantasies within the family. With hindsight, had I not hesitated, she may have experienced me as being able to bear her painful cris de coeur and to think safely and without fear about the deeper meaning of her remarks. Instead, I may have come across as colluding in the denial that was presented to the outside world by her family, that 'we are managing'.

Eva was the youngest of four in her immediate family, with a brother and two sisters. However, there was a sense both parents had a larger 'family in mind': her father had four siblings, her mother was one of seven and Eva had many cousins. Eva's brother was now away at college and her oldest sister, born with a profound and life-limiting condition, was being cared for at home with minimal respite, often, when her illness was at its worst, needing 24-hour nursing care. The family had developed a culture of denying the impact this had on them all. They received social care assistance but this was also perceived as critical and intrusive. Eva's other sister was just one year older, however, Eva was dismissive of any common ground, distancing herself further by choosing to attend a different secondary school from her sister.

In the absence of Eva's own thoughts about her unwittingly revealing comment, I pondered possible unconscious meanings. Did she desire the obliteration of 'one or more' of her siblings, and, if so, who should not be alive? Was it the sister whose care consumed the family's resources, something that might be unsayable, even unthinkable? Was it her brother, already on the way out? Or perhaps it was her closest sister, a rival; without her in the picture, Eva could be the 'perfect' girl for whom her parents would have room in their minds. Then again, Eva was the youngest, the fourth, and perhaps for her the solution was that she should not have been born. Did this fantasy solution aim to lighten their load or was it a furious and potentially fatal attempt to draw attention to their neglect of her and their inability to stop?

The work with Eva got off to a slow start. She incapacitated me with her silence, while at the same time I felt concern which I took as an indicator of hope. However, I found myself increasingly and at times frustratingly impotent in the room. If I tried to draw her out or derive meaning from what little she said, she would attack my attempt, splitting hairs or criticising its irrelevance, thus destroying my usefulness. It seemed impossible for Eva herself to acknowledge there was a problem, let alone participate in any solution proffered by school staff or support services. For a long time, she brought nothing of a personal nature. Socially isolated at school, the 'home in mind' of which she rarely spoke was so sparsely sketched as to seem utterly barren. She brought no evidence of play or relating, suggesting she almost entirely absented herself from family life.

All it seemed that was in our favour was consistency, with both of us able to stick with it over the longer term, for which we had the school's support. By the start of our second year, Eva was at last just about able to hear me speak about how difficult it was proving to think together, before throwing it back to me, saying it was 'my job' to find a way through. Latterly she was able to acknowledge, with a tinge of sadness, that if occasionally we did get to a place of speaking about something 'important' there was usually no time left to give it space. Though this acknowledgement of our process carried a sense of regret that time runs out in each session, it also explained the way she regulated our relating, and possibly with those at home too, as if the only safe way to admit feelings was just before cutting off contact. They were simply too powerful and dangerous to be allowed space.

Although it is possible that Eva's entrenched position would have presented challenges to any therapist, I think I was paralysed by my own unconscious resonances and corresponding denials. The theme of 'too many' with its disquieting subtext – which child 'shouldn't be there?' – and the denial of need ran through my own experience of family life. The fantasy of the barren family environment which had nothing to offer the child infused my work with Eva. Although I recognised that the function of depression might have been to dampen the savagery of intra-familial projections, I had, in this particular therapy setting, been fearful and avoidant of this just as I had been in the past in the context of my own family.

Conclusion

This book provides contributing therapists with the opportunity to speak openly about their own lives which has something of the quality of a presentation made at the culmination of some analytic trainings, not of a paper demonstrating clinical skill, but of the graduating trainee speaking about who they have become through their own analysis. Writing this chapter, and knowing it will have an audience, has been personally challenging and generated not a little resistance, manifested in repeatedly rethinking ethical and clinical considerations including the effect of my narrative on others, and of uncomfortable procrastination, not least for an initial period when I had yet to find a way to bring myself more fully into the story.

This has been a fertile process. Although I may have wished to control the content, it became more free-flowing along the way. Now that it is in the public domain, blind spots and all, those who read it might catch a glimpse of the unconscious at work: what slips through the cracks of my narrative and what I have left out or 'tidied up' is bound to be revealing. Writing this chapter is an attempt at a different sort of communication that marks a rite of passage for me. There is much to gain in owning our vulnerabilities and human frailties, and of taking note of how our experiences shape our practice and influence which theoretical texts we are most drawn to.

References

Barrie. J.M., (1906) *Peter Pan in Kensington Gardens.* London: Hodder and Stoughton.
Bates. H.E., (1958) *The Darling Buds of May.* London: Michael Joseph.
Coles. P., (2003) *The Importance of Sibling Relationships in Psychoanalysis.* London: Routledge.

Dolto. F., (1984) *L'Image inconsciente du corps*. Oaris: Le Seuil.

Dolto. F., in Hall. G., Hivernel. F., Morgan, S., (2009) *Theory and Practice in Child Psychoanalysis: An Introduction to the Work of Françoise Dolto*. London: Karnac Books Ltd. Chapter 5 "The Unconscious Image of the Body".

Evaristo. B., (2019) *Manifesto*. London: Penguin Books Ltd.

Lacan. J. & Sheridan. A., (1949) *The Mirror Stage as Formative of the Function of the I as Revealed in Psychoanalytic Experience*. 1st Edition. 17 May 2017. New York and London: W.W. Norton & Company.

Robertson. J. & Robertson. J., (1969) *John Aged Seventeen Months, for Nine Days in a Residential Nursery*. Film 43 mins John and Joyce Robertson, Robertson films.

Spock. B., (1957) *The Common Sense Book of Baby and Child Care*. 2nd Edition. New York: Duell Sloan and Pearce.

Truby King, F., (1923) *Feeding and Care of Baby*. London: Macmillan and Co.

Waller-Bridge. P., (2016) *Television Programme: Fleabag*. Comedy: BBC 3.

Winnicott. D.W. (ed.), (1967) Mirror role of mother and family in child development. In: *From Playing and Reality*. London: Tavistock Publications, pp. 149–160 (republished in 2005, New York: Routledge Classics).

Chapter 14

The search for belonging

An unfolding story

Mihoko Arayama

I was in my final year at a university in Japan working on my Master's dissertation in the library. When looking for some useful material, flicking through the pages of the journals, I came across an advertisement for a training in child psychotherapy in London. As someone always drawn to foreign countries, I found the full-page advert compelling. However, studying abroad sounded unrealistic and I only took a passing mental note of the course.

I chose psychology as my field of study when I was in my early twenties. Initially, my interest was in working with adolescents. My own difficult adolescence, during which I had wished there was someone who could listen to me non-judgmentally, was a strong influence in wanting to offer support to young people in difficulty. During my time at university, I was working part-time at a local child guidance centre to gain practical experience to support my academic research. Fortunately, I was offered many opportunities to work with children of different age ranges. They had a variety of issues, from learning difficulties to school refusal. The more I worked with those children and families, the more I wanted to explore their personality development especially the importance of their early experiences and its impact on their development. My interest gradually shifted from adolescence to earlier years, particularly infants' relationships with others, and grew stronger through my work experience with different cases. My understanding of mental functions brought to my attention disturbances in the early years, notably in relation to the infant–caregiver relationship, that could have a significant impact on the child's psychological development, staying with them through their life. This curiosity led me to focus on attachment theory which became the theme for my research at university.

After leaving university, I worked for a new service under a local educational authority that supported children with school refusal which had become a serious and growing issue in Japan. Although my interest had moved from adolescence to early infancy and I had spent more time working with infants and mothers during my studies, I settled into my role in supporting mainly secondary school pupils. This was a new provision in the area which my colleague and I launched from scratch. I was excited about it and enjoyed experiencing the service becoming well established and expanding.

DOI: 10.4324/9781003270447-15

Throughout this time the significance of children's early life and their relationships with their primary caregivers continued to inspire me to study more, which led me to psychoanalytic theory and object relations. The advertisement that I had come across in the university library three years earlier came back to me and I was now in the position to give it serious thought. Giving up a professional role that I had established in order to relocate to a country I had no connection with was by no means an easy decision. Conflicts and dilemmas competed with the compelling desire to learn more. Apart from leaving everyone I knew personally and professionally, I was proud of my job and I could have remained there. But my ambition to study abroad was strong and this brought me to the UK for further education and training in psychoanalysis. Over the years to follow, I completed my professional training to become a psychodynamic counsellor and psychotherapist for children and adolescents.

Although I continued to be drawn to focusing on very young children in infant–mother relationships, work opportunities again took me into secondary schools. Initially, I didn't question why I ended up seeing adolescents although I knew that my interest in infant and child development was very helpful in this work. It was only later on that I began to think about my own trajectory and what it meant. I reflected on my teenage years and my unconscious orientation in this work which motivated me to explore more deeply the influence of my life experience on my clinical practice. Thinking about the link between my past and present, I came to identify two key themes which have loomed large in my life – the world outside Japan and adolescence. Why was I so determined to study and work abroad and why did I gravitate towards adolescents when there were opportunities to pursue my interests and career taking a different path?

My backstory

I was born in Japan to Japanese parents. Life was simple and appeared straightforward in terms of social diversity. Growing up, I was not aware of any social classes, only nuanced differences in economic advantage. The country's geographic character as an island country and its historic isolationism have created a distinctive Japanese identity. 'Sakoku' (locked country) was a policy implemented in the 17th century that imposed limits to both migration and imports. It lasted for over 200 years. The politicians asserted over the years that Japan was a 'homogeneous society' and that the distinct nature of the country came from its isolationist ideology. Even after the second world war, this mentality was reinforced by the government offering centrally directed education and achieving one of the world's most equitable distributions of income that has had the longer-term effect of blurring class categories. This was the context in which I grew up. The majority of the population were average earners and defined themselves as middle class. They perceived their society as racially almost homogeneous and one rarely came across foreigners in daily life, although in reality there were some communities which consisted of other ethnic groups.

They were second or third-generation Korean and Chinese nationals who hid their identities in public to avoid racial discrimination. The nation's mentality that prioritised unity encouraged this collective sense of 'we are all the same'. Children learned very early on to conform with their peers which was reinforced through discipline. Seeking to stand out either through one's appearance or by holding differing opinions was thought to be morally wrong and to do so risked making one a target of criticism. Japanese people were frightened of being perceived as different and the social stigma this carried, leading most to suppress their authentic selves if they felt they might not fit in or match the image of who, or what, they were supposed to be. Even in the 1980s, the then prime minister commented publicly that ethnic diversity creates confusion and discord among the general public, sparking a dispute throughout the different political parties by declaring this. He stated that societies function best when people appear, think and act in a similar way, reflecting the majority Japanese view that government decisions are easier to make and implement in a homogeneous society (The Washington Post, 1986).

Being born, brought up and educated in this milieu, I wasn't allowed to be an exception to this rule. Nor was anyone else. However, since early childhood I was acutely aware of difference and of being different from those around me. Being the only person among my peers who had no siblings was enough to make me feel at odds with the others who had at least one brother or sister. But I had a more fundamental reason for being different. My father worked on a commercial ocean liner which meant he was away for six months of the year and then would be at home for the remaining half year. This made my life unique compared with my peers' families. It also affected aspects of my psychological development, as my father's frequent, and long absences made it impossible for me to experience a free-flowing relationship, characterised by an 'ongoing-ness' which could be taken for granted.

Nevertheless, there were some indications of an identification with my father in my childhood. From early on I presented as a tomboy, always wearing trousers and preferring to play with boys rather than other girls. I wanted to be a boy, to do the same things they did. With hindsight I imagine I wanted to be a powerful figure, to protect myself or/and my mother during the father's absence. Identifying with my father gave me, perhaps, a sense of safety. But at the same time I also enjoyed being protected by the boys when I would assume a girl's/daughter's role. I particularly remember one boy who would look after me as if he was a substitute for my absent father, giving me a sense of security.

I was also interested in things related to foreign countries. I especially liked Western TV programmes and often asked my mother the meanings of the foreign words which appeared on the packages of goods from abroad. My interest in other countries may have helped me to hold my father in mind as an internal object while he was away from home, mitigating some of the effects of his absences. But certainly as a toddler, my father's absences of up to six months at a time felt to me much longer. I couldn't remember him when he returned home.

There was another contribution to having the capacity to psychically hold on to my paternal object: my mother, who managed to sustain a good relationship with my father which supported and contained her during his absence. This enabled her to provide me with a fundamentally strong relationship that was essential for my healthy development. Maureen Marks writes about the mother's mediation of the father; the infant's experience of the father, whatever his actuality, is modified by how the mother presents the father to their baby, and this is determined by the mother's experience with her own father as mediated by her own mother (Marks, 2002). I assume that my mother's positive relationship with her own father greatly contributed to her ability to maintain a good relationship with her husband despite his physical absence. Marks also writes about the father as a second object. The earlier symbolising of fathers is thought to be due to the combined effect of fathers being absent more than mothers and of mothers facilitating the symbolising process by referring to the father in his absence. Thus, the mother contains the infant's anxieties about absence and the mental space this leaves so that it becomes possible for the child to think about the father as existing but absent. However, in my case, the repeated absences of my father and their influence on family life had an inescapable impact on my personality development which came to the surface later in my life.

My latency years were relatively peaceful. I stopped being a tomboy in a bid to hide my uniqueness and to fit in with my peers, encouraged by the stigma embedded in Japanese society against being different. By that time, my fatherless life with my mother for six months each year was well established. Concomitantly, my mother also seemed to be enjoying her time without her husband. She overtly expressed her disappointment when my father returned because of having to give up some of her social life due to my father being more anti-social. This obviously affected my daily life, too, restricting my freedom. The fact that I had two different lives, one with and one without my father, cast a shadow across my life. I, like my mother, split my life into 'good' and 'bad' according to whether my father was absent or present. Nevertheless, I managed to adjust to each situation and it seemed workable until puberty hit me and I entered adolescence.

It felt as if all that was left unprocessed from my infancy came back to trouble me in my adolescence. Firstly, I had an intense negative reaction to my femininity when puberty began. My body taking on a feminine shape shocked and even disgusted me and, as when I was a toddler, I profoundly wished to be a boy. While it took significant time to get used to this change, eventually I came to accept it. Laurence (2008) discusses the process of female puberty. As a girl healthily develops physically and mentally, her body prepares to take on the function of a potential container, foreshadowing motherhood to come. Among other things, this involves getting ready to give up the protection she has experienced until then; this is predicated on her having internalised a sense of security and protection. Her mind, at this time, also begins to develop the capacity for empathy and generosity. These changes are possible where the girl's relationship with her father has been good enough to enable her to internalise a primarily benign and constant paternal object (Laurence, 2008). Although my childhood didn't seem to be overtly damaging, there was an essential part that was missing, that should have provided the basis for a belief in a secure and stable world. This lack of that belief was felt intensely at this point in my adolescence and seems to have contributed to higher levels of anxiety and difficulty in accepting my puberty.

A few years later, my father retired from his work. That meant that he would never again be gone for six months at a time and instead stayed home the full calendar year. It was a huge and disturbing transition, one which felt intrusive to my peaceful life with my mother, let alone my own life. Both my mother and I had to mentally prepare for this in the knowledge that there was nothing we could do but accept the new circumstances. It was daunting: my first experience of living with my father every day without break – and I was a teenager. I had to work through what I had potentially missed out on – living in a triadic relationship with both parents, never having negotiated the Oedipus complex earlier due to my father's physical absence.

What I couldn't have anticipated was that my father chose to live independently of us, creating his own living space within the family house as if maintaining the lifestyle that he had had most of his life, in a cabin on the ship. This unintentionally helped preserve my phantasy of an exclusive bond with my mother. For this reason, at times, I felt my father's actual presence as a threat to life as I knew it. Britton (1998) discusses Oedipal illusions which take place when the reality and the facts (the parental relationship) are already known but their significance is unconsciously evaded and its nature not acknowledged by the child. These illusions provide a domain that is separate and free from the realities of the external world protecting the psyche from the phantasy of the Oedipal situation, which Britton says is present in normal development. The child oscillates between these two states of mind – 'illusionment' and 'disillusionment' as they adjust to Oedipal realities. However, when development is impinged on by an unsatisfactory reality, the illusion persists and slows down or even damages emotional development. Considering the characteristics of my relationship with my parents, I needed a longer period to navigate adolescent developmental task because my real circumstances allowed me to maintain a comfortable dyadic relationship with my mother. It reinforced an unhelpful 'good/bad' split represented by *'with my father'* and *'without him'*. My difficulty was both accepting the reality of my parents as a couple and being able to relinquish my belief in my psychic reality – thereby acknowledging the loss of my cosy intimacy with my mother – and integrating two different parts of my life. I struggled with this difficulty, acting out in response to it throughout my adolescence.

Perceiving parents as separate individuals who can no longer be seen as 'perfect' and who have their own life together seemed so unbearable to me that they became a target of my hatred. I became quite defiant against my parents and against authority in general while grappling with the search for my own identity. Once I had been afraid of being labelled as different because of societal pressures. And now I had become more conscious of my differences from others, and deliberately strove to be more unique. At the same time, I suffered from loneliness and tried to combat this by connecting to those who had similar interests and perspectives, all the while hampered by difficulties in finding words to express myself. As a consequence of the many clashes with my parents, I feared I had irretrievably lost their trust in me but in reality I found both of them were still there to support me.

The experience with my parents as a reunited couple provided me with the mental space to reflect on myself more objectively. From that point I gradually became able to grow emotionally, independent of my parents. This came with the emergence of a more trustful self that enabled me to think and decide for myself, whilst accepting my parents as separate, independent individuals with their own lives and their own histories. I accepted them as a parental couple, as my parents. Alongside my mother, my father eventually took a role in facilitating my emotional separation from my mother and provided me with a sense of security to better navigate the external world. This was another element in the process that enabled me to overcome the loss of what I had had and to explore external reality as an independent individual.

There are different aspects of myself which I have had to equally accept and integrate. One is a part that was cultivated in Japanese culture and the other that was shaped by the uniqueness of my family life and by my father who represented the world outside Japan. A product of this integration process was choosing psychology for my future career and eventually deciding to study and work abroad. Tellingly, the focus of my academic interests also shifted from the mother-infant dyadic relationship to the triadic structure which included a father, regardless of whether an actual, physical father is available in a child's life.

So, as I have tried to describe, my journey to becoming a psychotherapist working with adolescents was significantly influenced by my own struggles in adolescence. My search for myself and for the reason for my struggles led me into academic research and ultimately, to the choice of psychotherapy training.

Clinical work

I have been working with adolescents for nearly 30 years now. Most of my clients in Japan were living with both parents. However, it was usually only the mothers who sought help for their children, and there were few active paternal figures in their children's stories. I was fully aware of this but didn't pay much attention to its contribution to the children's mental health because I was so intently focused on mother–child relationships at that time. Once I moved to the UK, I soon noticed that the fathers of the majority of my clients were physically absent and that the children lived with their mothers as a sole parent either from the beginning of their lives or as a result of their parents' separation.

I have come across a number of children who have an intimate and intricate, often negative, relationship with their mothers. While able to express their more difficult feelings towards their father, they would soon back pedal, denying their impact to the point of repressing these at times overwhelming feelings, dismissing them by saying, 'But I don't care'. Such an imbalanced relationship with their parents has the potential to impact negatively on adolescents' mental health and wellbeing at a time when they are reworking developmental tasks tracking back to their infancy in order to find their own identity and achieve their independence, this time more realistically.

Many of my clients experience themselves as different from the majority of their peers. This is a characteristic of adolescence more generally but those who need psychological support find it much harder to negotiate these developmental tasks. In Japan, as I have mentioned, I was working with school refusal, a growing phenomenon in a society that doesn't easily understand the issue and has an entrenched prejudice against young people who do not conform with others. I was able to resonate with these 'outsiders' and shared their resentment and rebelliousness against the stubborn homogeneous mentality in Japan. It was an echo of what I had been feeling when I was a teenager: why do people need to be the same when we are all different? This identification with school refusers had an impact on my work, resulting in conveying to them that they were not doing anything wrong. On the contrary, they were simply caught up in a transitory developmental need to have a break from school to re-work something they had missed in the past.

As curious as it might seem, unlike many other Asian people here in London, including Japanese, I don't feel self-conscious about being different. This isn't only because of London's ethnic and cultural diversity but is also down to my experience of being the odd one out in a homogeneous society in Japan. Many young people brought up and living in London's multicultural society struggle to find their identities and also strive to fit in. Perhaps their experience of feeling different in such a diverse society is not so far removed from my sense of being an outsider in such a deeply conformist society that I grew up in. My struggle for an accepted identity has parallels with some of the young people I see.

The majority of my clients are second or third-generation immigrants to the UK, brought up within families where the adults have maintained the customs connected to their country of origin while they attend British schools and absorb the local culture. They often feel as if they are living simultaneously in two different dimensions. Younger children seem to naturally accept this reality but as they grow older, they begin to question which 'world' they wish to belong in. This context easily lends itself to value judgements, assigning aspects of each culture either 'good' or 'bad' and they struggle to negotiate between them. Although they would like to belong to one socio-cultural group, there is always an underlying mismatch that makes them feel there is no right fit for them, leaving them feeling alone and different from others.

I have seen many young people whose homes are not regarded as a comfortable place, a refuge for consolation and for recharging their emotional and mental energy. Instead, they have difficulties dealing with their circumstances and with their unprocessed emotions in relation to parents who, in their view, create these difficulties as well as confusion. Many of them unconsciously repress anger towards and sadness about their parents, acting out or manifesting mental health symptoms, for which they are referred to professionals like me. Concomitantly, despite their deprived circumstances, I am often impressed by some young people's resilience in never giving up their belief in their parents, perhaps indicating an acceptance of the denied parts of themselves.

One client, Iman, aged 15 when referred to me, had been feeling distant from her father who was usually busy with his work and seldom stayed with his family. She said she hated him because he privileged her older brothers at her expense, believing this was due to the family's ethnic background which accorded males superior status. She felt close to her mother and expected her to understand her difficult position. But it was a complicated relationship primarily because of her mother's apparent collusion with the cultural norms. Iman had repressed her dissatisfaction with her parents until she became a teenager at which point she began to really struggle. Her referral followed an emotional outburst at school. She revealed to me the extent to which she had been distancing herself from more difficult feelings since she was very young by trying to do well and be a good daughter in the family, particularly in comparison with her brothers. Iman also managed to come across as fine in public by denying all her problems. She had been quite capable of appearing stable until, at age fifteen, she felt unable to control herself anymore.

Iman required considerable time before she could be honest with herself and express feelings and thoughts that were less comfortable to own. Her acknowledgement of her difficulties and their detrimental effects on her mental wellbeing was a helpful step. She began working towards becoming more aware of what she was feeling and finding the words to express this. Gradually, Iman became more able to be in touch with the painful emotions that had been pushed down and denied for many years. Her powerful feelings about her parents, particularly towards her father, were palpable to me. At the same time, I was also conscious of her need to go through this difficult process in order to become more stable and whole. I was able to co-create a relationship with her within which she could freely express the many emotions she was experiencing. Having gone through this re-working process, with time, Iman was able to see her parents differently. She grew to accept that they had their own lives and that their behaviours and attitudes were based on both their personal experiences and cultural circumstances. She saw them as a couple interacting with each other and was able to accept being excluded from aspects of their relationship. This understanding paved the way for better communication with each parent and for forgiveness for their treatment of her in the past. She also started regarding her ethnic background with more respect and saw ways of incorporating it into her own cultural background cultivated in the UK. The pride she developed around her ethnicity sat alongside her desire to become a professionally independent young woman, rather than subject to male power. Her confidence in herself and her future grew exponentially as did her capacity to manage her anxiety at stressful times. By the time we ended, she had come to recognise and accept both parents and her ethnic background as parts of herself by integrating them into her own identity, becoming a more confident, independent person.

Working with Iman reminded me of my susceptibility to feeling powerful emotions when clients' narratives involve missing fathers and closeness with their mothers. Strong resonances also emerge when working with clients from different cultural backgrounds, especially when conflicts between their ethnicity and British culture feature or they try to hide their uniqueness. I can sense how poignantly they feel the lonely struggle of finding a sense of belonging. The echoes with my life experience enable me to empathise while being alert to over-identification with these young people. Understanding my own past helps me to be aware of the importance of countertransference and also to notice the clients' potential ability to progress when I see their hidden hope – that of never wanting to give up their parents.

Children from different ethnic groups and complicated family backgrounds can find their diversity brings up conflicting feelings and they can face additional challenges in shaping their identity, especially if they belong to more than one social group. For them, the integration of these different parts and self-states is a key factor for their healthy development. They then become able to accept their reality which can mitigate their anger and betrayal about their circumstances 'letting them down' and avoid a sense of the self being split into multiple parts. Because of my own struggles in adolescence to find a place and identity that fit, supporting my young clients by offering them a thinking space feels particularly fulfilling.

Conclusion

As a psychotherapist, I understand that my life history has influenced my present self and career choice. My background, pivotal childhood experiences and adult life events contribute to my personality development, professional functioning, choice of theoretical positions and clinical techniques. Therapists' subjectivity is a part of us, of our way of hearing, processing, and interacting with our clients. And the dynamics between therapist and client are always driven by the nature of the intersubjective experience between them, determining the tone of the therapeutic relationship.

In psychotherapy training, we learn of the importance of self-awareness as a tool to establish healthy boundaries with our clients and to distinguish between transference and countertransference. Being self-aware enables the therapist to discriminate between what belongs to them and what belongs to their clients.

For this purpose, I have undergone personal analysis for a considerable period, which provided a wholly unique opportunity to reflect intensively on myself and my history.

But sharing my life experience with fellow therapists over the years was a different matter. I found it challenging and, in the face of my resistance to the process, had to summon courage and determination to revisit emotionally difficult experiences from the past. My resistance resurfaced at the prospect of writing this chapter. However, the experience offered me another valuable opportunity for self-analysis, enabling me to look more deeply, reminding me of the experience of my personal analysis – a process that is still actively at work in my mind when I reflect on myself, giving me a better understanding of myself as well as those I work with and relate to.

References

Britton, R. (1989). The Missing Link: Parental Sexuality in the Oedipus Complex. In: Britton, R., Feldman, M. and O'Shaughnessy, E. (Eds). *The Oedipus Complex Today* (pp. 83–102). London: Karnac.

Britton, R. (1998). *Belief and Imagination: Explorations in Psychoanalysis*. London: Routledge.

Burgess, J. (1986). *Japanese Proud of Their Homogeneous Society*. Washington, DC: The Washington Post.

Etchegoyen, A. (2002). Psychoanalytic Ideas about Fathers. In: Trowell, J. and Etchegoyen, A. (Eds). *The Importance of Fathers: A Psychoanalytic Re-evaluation* (pp. 84–96). East Essex: Brunner-Routledge.

Kuchunk, S. (Ed) (2014). *Clinical Implications of the Psychoanalyst's Life Experience: When the Persona Becomes Professional*. New York: Routledge.

Lawrence, M. (2008). *The Anorexic Mind. The Tavistock Clinic Series*. London: Karnac.

Marks, M. (2002). Letting Fathers In. In: Trowell, J. and Etchegoyen, A. (Eds). *The Importance of Fathers: A Psychoanalytic Re-evaluation* (pp. 84–96). East Essex: Brunner-Routledge.

Waddell, M. (2018). *On Adolescence: Inside Stories. The Tavistock Clinic Series*. London: Karnac.

Chapter 15

The meaning of home

The loss of the 'motherland' and how this shapes the formation of identity

Martina Nalesso

I was born in Italy and grew up there as an only child. During my childhood and my teenage years the northern part of Italy where my family resided was very much white demographically and the vast majority of the population was Italian. My neighbours were white Italians, my schoolmates were white Italians, and my teachers were white Italians. It was a completely different, homogeneous world in comparison to the multicultural society that Italy has become. In those days, Italians all spoke the same basic language yet with different accents and dialects but with the knowledge that we could all understand each other. Therefore, the idea that the world was made up of people with different cultural backgrounds, races, languages, religions, and colours was something I never gave much consideration to when I was a child. I didn't reflect on what it meant that my father was born in Belgium to Italian parents and lived there up until the age of 12 as he never spoke about his early years.

In fact, throughout his life, my father denied his Belgian identity. Perhaps there was an unconscious block around thinking about his nationality and what this might signify. Although I was curious about it and fascinated too, I dared not ask him questions about his childhood as I unconsciously registered an unspoken message to steer clear of it. It was simply never discussed in the family. All I knew was that my father's childhood was characterised by painful events which I now see had left him with unprocessed trauma which included issues around his identity. My father passed away more than 15 years ago which means many questions about his childhood remain unanswered. After his death, I went to visit the place where he was born and grew up, a small town just outside Namur where a large Italian community has settled and has been living for generations. Over the years, the place has evolved in different ways including changing its name. It was not possible to meet any relatives there as many of them, like my father, had also passed away.

Historically, Belgium is a country that has seen great waves of immigration. In the years soon after the Second World War when my grandparents moved there, Belgium recruited more than a million mine workers from all over Europe. My grandfather was one of them. In its more recent history, it has encountered divisions over differences of language and of unequal economic development.

DOI: 10.4324/9781003270447-16

A far-reaching series of reforms since the 1970s set the scene for the creation of three regions, each with its own official language: Flanders (Dutch-speaking) in the north, Wallonia (French-speaking) in the south, where my father was from, and bilingual Brussels in the middle. There is also a German-speaking population residing along the border with Germany. Nowadays, Belgium comprises many communities – Turkish, Moroccan, Italian, French, and Dutch – contributing to the country's cultural richness and diversity.

My impression of Belgium is of a nation without a clearly defined identity, lacking a sense of shared values or national pride. This has led me to think about my father's identity and, in turn, my own as an Italian now living in the UK. It has caused me to wonder whether my decision to move abroad had something to do with an intergenerational trauma that I carry within me which takes the form of a shadow in my psyche, as was the case with my father. Perhaps my need to relocate links with trying to make sense of my father's family experiences and to work through some of the challenges that he was never able to voice and understand. Consciously and willingly going through the process of losing what was familiar to me by jumping into the unknown when I moved first to Spain and then the UK meant that I could somehow put myself in my father's shoes and grieve what he never managed to mourn. I have always had the impression that my father found the separation from Belgium, and from the part of the family that he left behind when he moved to Italy, overwhelming for most of his life. Contrary to my father, moving abroad has given me the opportunity to grow and evolve and has offered me a sense of freedom that my father never experienced because his poignant memories and unresolved losses kept him trapped inside. My father did not have the emotional support from his family to grieve the losses involved, but he (and my mother) gave me the kind of love and encouragement which enabled me to go on a journey on my own and experience the physical and emotional separation from my parents and my motherland. I embrace the fact that I might represent for my family a way to process their unconscious need of making sense of past histories. It is a privilege to be able to do so.

I was always disappointed with my father for not teaching me French, which he spoke outside of the home for the first 12 years of his life. Intuitively, I felt the need to learn the language perhaps as a way of getting closer to him, to get to know that closed-off, mysterious side of him and to connect with the part of me that is somehow emotionally linked to Belgium. My father declined to formalise his Belgian nationality and tried hard to shed any hint of a French accent when pronouncing Italian words. By the time I was born, when my father was 27, he could speak perfect Italian but could not write with the same fluency and would get visibly upset when spelling mistakes were pointed out: maybe they were a reminder of his Belgian self, the part of his identity that he had tried so hard to leave behind. To me, this was a contradiction: he had been born in Belgium, so he wasn't completely Italian. It felt as if the part of his life linked to Belgium had to be erased.

My father left Belgium when he was in his early adolescence. Moving on from that country may have also felt like leaving childhood behind and beginning the transition into young adulthood. This could have given him the opportunity to create a new identity, forgetting about his Belgian self by avoiding speaking in French, choosing instead to communicate in Italian. He made new friendships with Italian peers which probably gave him a different sense of self and may have been empowering. Italy for my father was his motherland but also a foreign country. His need to build connections with Italian people and learn their language with its pronunciation, idioms, and dialects had the function of making him feel accepted and formed the basis for establishing his Italian identity. By feeling that he belonged to a place and a culture, he was probably less likely to experience stereotypes, racial slurs, and ethnic jokes, all things that I believe my father was exposed to when he was living in Belgium. As Gray (1996) suggests, the need to belong to a group can also be seen as a regressive attempt at re-creating a sense of merging or 'participation mystique' that can be seen in the mother–infant bond which influences groups' behaviour. Groups can re-establish a sense of belonging and safety that was originally experienced by the child in the symbiotic relationship with the mother making the individual feel omnipotent again. They can provide a sense of direction and refuge for those who have difficulties working on their individuation process. My father was never able, or emotionally ready, to use either of his two languages, Italian or French, to tell his story. If he had, he might have been able to distance himself from the traumas of his early years which may have allowed for a deeper, more meaningful connection with his own history and for the development of a stronger and healthier sense of self. As Pennebaker (as cited in Music, 2017) says, using words, especially shifting from the first pronoun (I) to the third person (he/she) or 'we' statements, is an aspect of affect regulation and can help the individual make sense of their internal states enabling them to manage overwhelming emotions. My father did not have this ability as I believe that feelings of shame, guilt, and perhaps fear of being hurt again where too intense to allow him to look more deeply into his past. Instead, he spent most of his life re-enacting aspects of his past, often in self-destructive ways. Only when he was nearing the end of his life and he knew that I was interested in becoming an art psychotherapist, did he show some willingness and readiness to talk about his feelings and was open to the idea of accessing emotional support. It was, regrettably, too late as he passed away soon after.

Looking back, and from what I now know, it is as if my father lived in a state of grief all his life. First and foremost, he was grieving the loss of his 'Great Mother Italy' by identifying with his mother's feeling of profound loss of home. When the family moved back to Italy, he was faced with the loss of his grandmother who stayed in Belgium and who represented the 'Great Mother' in the family unconscious: she was the person who could keep the family together. He was also grieving the loss of his adoptive homeland Belgium and with it, his Belgian Self.

His family left for Belgium at a time when Italy had few economic opportunities and was therefore not the symbolic 'good breast' mother country, bountiful and giving, but the depleted or withholding one. When the family eventually decided to move back to Italy, the better future they had hoped for there turned out to be an illusion. Italy was not the 'good object' that my father and his family had wished for. Belgium, on the other hand, had the quality of an ambivalent 'adoptive mother' which gave my father's family a degree of financial security but also some painful experiences, including my granddad's illness. He contracted silicosis when working for a short period of time as a miner and that was the main reason for relocating to Italy. I suppose that, especially for my granddad, the return to Italy was felt and imagined as a comforting return to a warm, safe, and welcoming place. However, relocating back to Italy marked the crumbling of the family's mythologising of Italy as 'Great Mother' and with it, the collapse of all hope for a better future that Italy must have represented in their collective mind. So, my father had to grieve once again the loss of the internalised good object, the 'motherland'. He perpetuated throughout his life the splitting of his identity without ever being able to fully integrate the contrasting aspects of his Belgian and Italian parts. My father lived his Belgian identity as a 'borrowed' or 'transitory' identity which would have stayed in his unconscious, representing something perhaps shameful or unnameable tied up with notions of betrayal and abandonment linked to for-saking the 'true motherland', Italy.

My father's experience of living abroad settled in the unconscious of our family history. It is no surprise to me that, in my 20s, I decided to leave Italy. As I have mentioned, a primary drive, although I may not have been fully aware of it at the time, was that I needed to make sense of what happened to my father by exposing myself to similar experiences of dislocation and loss. Living first in Spain and then in the UK, I had to learn two new languages, become ac-customed to new lifestyles, get used to forming new kinds of relationships and different expectations within them, and find new ways of using an acquired language to communicate in and out of the therapeutic setting. I also had to face my own assumptions and stereotypes as well as what I have come to see as my internalised racism. Additionally, from time to time, I have experienced myself as the object of stereotypes and assumptions and a container for the disowned visible and invisible differences of others.

For me as an only child, moving abroad meant loosening the ties of dependency with my mother, both physically and symbolically. The memories of my mother and the memories of the 'Great Mother Italy' have now become intertwined in my unconscious. The soul of my place of origin with its colours, sounds, climate, customs, and traditions is intimately connected to my mother's colourful sides, vocal tones, affection, habits, and ways of being. When I speak with her on the phone, the sound of her voice with its particular pitch and rhythm takes me back to my childhood, to those places where I spent most of my time with her. I remember the smells, the colours, and the sounds of those places too. No matter what we talk about, images of my childhood surface when I hear her voice.

During the first year of my life, my mother spent all of her time with me. Because of this, I developed my language skills very quickly. By the age of around ten months, I could say my full name and by 12 months, I could construct long sentences even though not all the words were clearly pronounced. However, when I was older and experienced some very distressing events in primary school where I had a teacher who was unreasonably harsh and used physical punishment as a form of discipline, I couldn't draw on emotional support from either of my parents. This may reflect what happens in families when earlier pain and loss have not been fully processed and denial or repression becomes the modus operandi. Without the vocabulary to describe what I was experiencing, I was not able to use language to express how I was feeling. As a consequence, I shut down. In common with my father, I did not have a language to tell my story and could not distance myself from the traumatic events I had experienced. Instead, as with many children and young people I see today in school-based psychotherapy sessions, my distress was expressed non-verbally through physical ailments such as stomach aches and headaches.

Training in art psychotherapy necessitated building an emotional vocabulary in order to better understand myself, to give voice to my life experiences and to understand the way in which the unconscious manifests itself. And I undertook this in English, a language that I do not share with my mother. Looking back, I now wonder if my mother has been grieving the loss of her daughter all these years and the loss of the possibility to have a common mother tongue, a common language that the two of us can use to express and share our deepest emotions. However, that early bond which my mother and I established when I was an infant is an enduring one, forming the root of my attachment with her. My sense of her as a secure base is linked to the connection that I feel with Italy: a welcoming, warm, and lively place in my unconscious, a place to which I am always happy to return.

My acculturation process to Britishness and the English language was long and not always easy. I went through different phases, including denigrating my own country (perhaps best understood as a compensation for lost identity) alternating with denigration of the new country (a form of anger over all that had been lost), as well as vacillating between rejection of the new country's culture and a turning away from my own culture and language. For instance, initially, I did not want to have Italian friends in London, and I used to avoid reading in Italian, briefly labelling it as 'boring' (not as exciting or as challenging as reading in English). Just as my father tried hard to rid himself of his French accent, I too worked on toning down my Italian accent but with only limited success. While I inherited my father's shame of having an accent, there is no denying that I do, and I have now accepted that it is part of who I am. Frequently, people cannot place my accent, an experience which leaves me feeling in between identities. This is not the case in Italy where I have a Northern accent and people recognise where I come from because of it, something which gives me a comfortable sense of belonging. As Giselle China (in Zarbafi & Wilson, 2021) writes, an accent denotes difference of emotional and cultural thinking and perceptions. Having an imperceptible accent might be used as a defence against the feeling of otherness and might fulfil the need to 'fit in' which then creates the false assumption that a language spoken correctly indicates that the person knows and understands the culture of the country.

My accent stimulates curiosity in people who straightaway ask me where I'm from to strike up a conversation, unaware that such a question is a way of making me feel different. Especially in the current political climate (post-Brexit) I wonder about the reaction British people may have when I say that I am Italian, despite the fact that it is usually positive. My adoptive British 'motherland' has taken on the quality of an ambivalent mother. The UK has given me many exciting and interesting opportunities both personally and professionally, but the physical distance from my family can, at times, make me perceive this country as 'unemotional' in my mind.

When I started my therapy training, for some time I was the only non-native English speaker in the group. Communicating with other students was hard especially outside lecture hours when the use of language was less formal, and it took me a while to understand the way British people express themselves verbally and non-verbally. At times, I can still find myself 'lost in translation' and in those moments, language becomes a barrier blocking group cohesion and hindering my sense of belonging. I had to develop new thought pathways and affects in order to communicate more freely and comfortably with British people. Also, Italian people are famous around the world for using their body in a very expressive way in social interactions. My 'Italian Self' has had to constantly remind my 'British Self' that personal space is different in this country. In Italy, we do not have an equivalent personal space but rather a shared collective space. Physical boundaries are different, and we usually breach them when we communicate, such as with frequent touch.

These conflicting emotions have now been understood and integrated. I have accepted the fact that when I am in the UK, I have to 'perform' new social roles and ways of being. While I feel I need to renounce some aspects of my Italian self (e.g., humour, spontaneity, fluidity of speech and movement) both in and outside therapy sessions, unlike my parents and perhaps most of their generation I have had the good fortune to gain an emotional vocabulary and the ability to organise my experiences into a fuller narrative without a compelling need to disguise or disown parts of who I am. Being able to talk about my own life experiences also makes me feel more connected to other people. As Davis (2014) suggests by sharing our experiences we build bridges allowing us to feel closer to the Other who otherwise can be felt as alien.

I constantly need to reorganise my identity; even when I go back to Italy and I feel 'myself' (that is, less self-conscious and freer in my communication), my British Self is always present and does not want to be forgotten. So, for instance,

I find myself punctuating my sentences with English words and saying 'thank you' and 'please' repeatedly, much to the amusement of my Italian friends! I often feel caught between two cultures and languages, but it is no longer an uncomfortable place to occupy. Overall, I can relate to what Natsu Hattori (in Zarbafi & Wilson, 2021) says when she writes that sometimes the change of country and identity is 'the making' of immigrants. Through my immigration experience, I had the opportunity to explore and reinvent myself and I could challenge some of the closeminded views that are present in some layers of the Italian society. The UK has helped me become more flexible in my thinking and ways of being. In The Babel of the Unconscious, Amati-Mehler and his colleagues (as cited in Davis, 2014), explore this issue in depth. They suggest that mastering a new language after childhood can offer the opportunity to develop new affective experiences, side-stepping some unconscious childhood conflicts, and can provide the opportunity to use the language for new social functions that can also be linked to a different social status.

In my work as a psychotherapist based in schools, I often wonder if I can really attune myself to my clients and understand their thoughts and feelings when I am not speaking in my mother tongue. As the term suggests, language most commonly develops within the mother–infant relationship and is therefore imbued with an emotional charge. I am aware of the fact that I have a less expansive vocabulary in English and that I can make mistakes when I speak and write. This gives me a sense of insecurity – inferiority even – as well as estrangement. Having to communicate in English can also be mentally draining and when I am particularly tired, I tend to speak in Italian or get confused between the two languages. This is known in linguistics as 'code switching' or 'language alternation' which is common among multilingual people. In my case, creating sentences that contain both Italian and English tap into my need to express and feel my sense of cultural identity and belonging and might also represent that side of myself that wants to differentiate from society at large.

I have noticed that I use English rather than Italian to express difficult emotions, perhaps as a way of distancing myself from the pain that some words may trigger in me. I can also have bodily sensations when I communicate difficult emotions in Italian, their intensity varying depending on who I am talking to. The prosody of the two languages is also different as patterns of rhythm and sound are connected to levels of intimacy. And the choice of words is linked to degrees of intimacy too. For instance, in my personal therapy I have chosen to work with British therapists which I believe has helped me in dealing with some more difficult emotions as I could express them verbally without the threat of being overwhelmed by them. John Clare (as cited in Zarbafi & Wilson, 2004), amongst others, has noted how for some clients the use of the acquired language in personal therapy, can provide them with some psychic space that can enable their need to verbalise the unspeakable, including the loss of the mother country. Paradoxically, while my emotional vocabulary is richer in English than in Italian it is less emotionally invested. When the mother tongue is charged with heavy emotions, the use of a foreign language can bring the ambiguity which enables distance and perspective (ibid.). It is only the language of the unconscious (artmaking and dreams) that allows me to explore my deeper feelings in an emotional but not overwhelming way. For these reasons I consider myself a British therapist. As I trained in London and undertook personal therapy in English, I am not certain I would be able to find the right words in Italian to support my clients.

The processes I have been through in developing an emotionally informed therapeutic language to work in have been aided by my first training in art psychotherapy. Using visual language as a vehicle for expression came into its own when I worked with a secondary school student who was a selective mute. Isabel had been adopted as a young child from a Spanish-speaking South American country and had spent her formative years in Italy as her adoptive parents were Italian. On moving to London and joining a large secondary school, at 12 years of age, she found speaking to adults unbearable. The use of the art materials allowed her to work through some of the primal experiences of separation and abandonment that Isabel experienced as an infant. The non-verbal language of art gave her the opportunity to give voice to unconscious feelings that Isabel wouldn't have been able to verbalise in other ways. Her creative use of playdough and water movingly reminded me of an intrauterine life and of the birth experience. Using these materials facilitated the expression of what I believe was a painful and confusing time for her. Isabel couldn't give words to that experience, not only because she was too young to consciously remember it, but also because it is likely she had to suppress the side of herself that was connected to her birth mother and her experiences in her country of origin. Growing up she had to adapt to her new life in Italy and subsequently in the UK. She had to learn Italian and English and forget the sound of her mother tongue. The language spoken by her birth mother would have lost meaning and symbolic power in her psyche, or perhaps had never had the chance to take root.

Moving to London on the cusp of her teen years seemed to have triggered a re-enactment of the first important separation that Isabel experienced as an infant. Although I had the option of speaking Italian to Isabel which might have opened up verbal conversation with her, it felt important that I respected her silence. I had the feeling that some pre-object and primitive states of mind, when the baby has a symbiotic relationship with the mother, had been re-enacted in my relationship with Isabel. She seemed to use her persistent silence and the art materials to work through her early relationship with her birth mother. Maybe the fact that I was Italian, which she knew, facilitated our relationship and her ability to trust me straight away. A sense of 'feeling at home' because I could speak the same language that she and her adoptive parents spoke, allowed Isabel to feel I could understand her.

I also had the impression that Isabel was using me as a supporting ego. Through her silence I was perhaps experiencing something akin to what she had been through as a baby, and I could feel the passiveness of her early experiences.

The silence in the room required me to be alert and reflective all the time so I could verbalise what was going on in the sessions and what I was perceiving might have gone on inside Isabel. There was a creative quality in Isabel's silence that seemed to enable access to early psychic stages of ego development. Isabel also needed to know that I was mentally and emotionally present; this seemed to allow her to feel safe enough to start the unconscious process of separating from her birth mother. This meant getting in touch with and starting to grieve the loss of her mother as well as all the emotional and cultural aspects of identity that a mother carries within herself. Isabel's silent creative expression combined with the words I used to make sense of what she was expressing, always in English but with the accent and cadences of Italian, may have given her the feeling that she could gradually and safely bring to the surface repressed fragments of history. Through the artmaking, the silences, and my carefully chosen interpretations, Isabel started a process of integrating the different parts of herself. It seemed this gave her a sense of freedom from an internal 'silencing' which may have been linked to felt memories of a long absent birth mother, memories too raw to give words to. The experience of being in a very particular kind of dyadic relationship with me gradually took hold; who I am, and what I represented to Isabel both consciously and unconsciously seemed an integral component of the therapeutic relationship, a relationship that always draws so powerfully and uniquely from both the therapist's and the client's unconscious subjectivity and that creates what Odgen (1994) calls the analytic third. Over time, Isabel showed an increased ability to communicate verbally with the adults around her and started to feel less anxious and more confident with herself.

My background and my family experiences may have played their part in enabling Isabel both to find and create what she needed within herself. It is difficult to put into words the layered communications, verbal and non-verbal, visual and felt, that together generate the quality of any therapeutic relationship. With Isabel, the lost birth mother, the lost first language and the experiences of re-locating to a new and unknown country all found expression within and without. Discovering the hidden parts of ourselves, even though it can be highly painful and distressing at times, allows for the possibility of authentic expression and experience as well as helps to reduce the intensity of individual or collective trauma that can otherwise be passed down the generations. Finding a way to share our painful and often confusing past experiences can be very liberating and transformative. The way we use language, the choice of words, the emotional resonance that they produce within ourselves, the ability to share our life experiences with the Other, all make it possible for trauma to be expressed, understood, and overcome. My family's past will always be part of who I am, but I now feel more at ease working on the many layers of unspoken and unprocessed events that have been left me with by my ancestors. I will continue to be curious about this heritage and accept that the intergenerational transmission of emotions is unavoidable but also manageable. If we own it and explore it, it can enrich our lives.

References

Davis M. (2014). *Language and Connection in Psychotherapy*, London: Rowman & Littlefield.

Gray R.M. (1996). *Archetypal Explorations. An Integrative Approach to Human Behaviour*, London: Routledge.

Music G. (2017). *Nurturing Natures. Attachment and Children's Emotional, Sociocultural and Brain Development*, Oxon: Routledge.

Odgen T.H. (1994). The Analytic Third: Working with Intersubjective Clinical Facts. *International Journal of Psycho-Analysis*, 75:3–19.

Zarbafi A., Wilson S. (2021). *Mother Tongue and Other Tongues. Narratives in Multilingual Psychotherapy*, Oxfordshire: Phoenix Publishing House.

Chapter 16

Parenting a child through a life-threatening illness

Then and now

Marta Alonso

When it was proposed that I write about my dual experience as a mother who was faced with supporting my child through a life-threatening illness, and as a therapist who has worked with children and mothers who have gone through something similar, I felt conflicted. Would I be able to stay true to the raw and almost indescribable heightened sensibility that defined my world at that time? Or would I inevitably betray my 'mother-part' by trying to articulate my lived story from a more rational, psychoanalytic perspective; perhaps, even defending against going back in time to the emotional reality of my life then?

Somehow the archetype of the wounded healer helped me to reflect on, and make more sense of, these two aspects of my identity. It reminded me that re-processing life-changing experiences and continuing to try to bring unconscious material into awareness could help me in my work as a therapist, especially with families going through a similar experience.

A child's serious illness seeps into the life of everyone in the family, bringing with it a dawning of the real possibility of death and the fear that accompanies this, along with the crushing reality of the lack of control any of us have over life itself. Although recovery and even cure can happen, anticipatory grief will inevitably reverberate in the life of the child and those around them. Life is turned upside down. The possibility of surviving one's own child feels unbearably painful and even to think this thought seems to risk 'making it happen'. What does one do with this reality? Can a mother hold the whole picture in mind, including all the potential outcomes, in the way that a 'good enough' therapist would aim to? Or is it asking too much? But who is better placed, if not the mother, to hold this actuality and its emotional resonance on behalf of the child? Or does a concept like this simply become irrelevant when confronted with having to survive the anxieties each day, while simultaneously keeping hope alive not just for oneself but for the child and the rest of the family?

Death and its inevitability are downplayed in our contemporary world. We are regularly fed reports of continual advances in medical research and breakthroughs in discovering treatments for what used to be terminal illnesses. This, combined with the influence of the pharmaceutical world which is driven in

DOI: 10.4324/9781003270447-17

part by market forces, offers us a false sense of mastery over life and death. A more recent shift in our capacity to acknowledge the reality of death has occurred in the context of the global pandemic which has shaken everyone's certainty and sense of control.

When the national lockdowns resulted in school therapists shifting their way of working to support parents and children remotely, I was aware of similar responses to those I had experienced during my daughter's treatment when uncertainty, along with the tides of unconscious fears and anxieties, made looking into the future or the past a source of difficult questions and extreme feelings. At that time as a family, we were forced to take refuge in living in the moment and staying there, one day at a time. And during periods of lockdown I saw echoes of this pull into the present as something shared by all. Looking back at the time of my daughter's illness stirred feelings of grief for a time of greater freedom and health while not knowing what the pandemic might bring made projecting into the future uncomfortable too.

Proximity to death sheds light on our need for a degree of control and predictability in the everyday but also puts life into sharp perspective. Our previous daily worries suddenly appear trivial while sources of support and emotional nourishment such as hospitals, schools, government aid, communities, and families come to the fore. If facing our own mortality is a task perpetually put off, how equipped can we possibly be to deal with the prospect of losing a child? Such an occurrence is unthinkable for any parent but also a great shock for siblings as well as all those in the family's wider circles. I was fortunate in being able to rely on the strength and involvement of my extended family throughout my daughter's illness, confirming the power of close bonds of attachment in containing fear and pain.

For a mother, the mere thought of losing her child can feel simply unbearable. Carrying the weight of knowing that my child would need to go through an invasive medical treatment which would affect her wellbeing left me in unknown territory, an empty space of raw terror, where the only salvation was building hope out of nothing, as there were no guarantees that the treatment would succeed. I remember the shock I felt on the day of diagnosis. I felt fear creeping into my mind symbolically in the shape of an old song I know which describes a tragic story, just like the one I was trying very hard to avoid considering. The only tool I had to fight this was owning that fear and then creating a counter narrative, which I repeated like a mantra, to keep me afloat. It is now clear to me how vital it was to fully acknowledge to myself the existence of terror. I had to let the unconscious fear of death become conscious instead of splitting it off or denying it. It was only after getting in touch with all of my feelings, however painful, that I was able to gain some control over my mind.

However, some of the unconscious feelings took longer to surface. I remember my surprise at the initial meeting with the radiologist when she said, 'First of all, I want you to know that this is not your fault'. I felt confused by her reassurance, as the possibility of being responsible for my daughter's brain cancer was not something I had considered at that time. Months later I found myself repeatedly wondering if I could pinpoint the precise moment when that first cancer cell started abnormally dividing, irrational though this was. Trying to identify a specific time when this may have happened – perhaps in an attempt to build a coherent narrative of our story – brought an acute sense of responsibility and a taste of guilt. I now understand that it can be easier to feel guilty and therefore 'in control' rather than giving in to the truth that we will never be able to keep our children from all the possible dangers in life, however hard we try to protect them.

Guilt is bound to make itself felt in everyone who is close to someone seriously ill. This feeling is one that we quickly repress as it can be intolerable to imagine that we may be in some way responsible for a family member's disease, illogical though this is. More recently, we have all experienced this during the global pandemic. Any of us could potentially carry the virus and unknowingly pass it on to a loved one or someone who may be vulnerable, causing serious illness and even death. This brings to mind the sense of blame and guilt recorded during the time of the Black Plague with some suggesting it was God's way of punishing disobedient Catholics or that it originated in children who disobeyed their parents. Our belief system or worldview shapes the meanings we give reality, especially in times of crisis when we seek explanations, trying to fill in the gaps of an otherwise inexplicable tragedy.

In *Armfuls of Time: The Psychological Experience of the Child with a Life-Threatening Illness* (1986), Sourkes points out that the child's concrete thinking does not easily permit the concept of randomness to have any meaning, and so it is important to explore the sense they make of their illness. Also, although 'treatment' is a word which, within a medical context, we have positive associations with, it is difficult for the child to understand its meaning. Treatment can seem to be a form of punishment in a child's eyes and might make them act over-compliantly in the hope that good behaviour will be rewarded with less pain. However, the child may fall into the opposite trap: believing that they must have brought the illness on by 'being bad', they start acting out as a way of releasing their stress and anxiety. Both positions can be seen as manifestations of the child's belief system around their illness and need to be watched out for.

More recently my work with one of the primary school children I see brought to the fore the importance of responding sensitively to different cultures and beliefs in therapy. Akyra had experienced a recent tragic death in her family while, at the same time, bearing witness to her mother's long-term illness. She started thinking her family was 'cursed' and that she was 'bad' with 'demons inside'. Her way of making sense of these experiences might reflect aspects of her religious upbringing but felt an obstacle to her development and grieving process. In this case I was able to help Akyra without challenging her religious beliefs. I achieved this by reframing her thinking and building a different narrative where she was not responsible for the tragedies in her life.

When our mind meets the unimaginable, there is an overriding need to find meaning. In the middle of my then-broken life, I could observe my thoughts linking together events, dates, details – mere random facts – in order to create a constellation of events which would, if I tried hard enough, (or so I thought), fall into a coherent narrative, even if I could see how non-sensical this all was. It may be akin to how an individual might experience a psychotic crisis with objects and events being interpreted in a symbolic manner in the service of creating a story that can 'hold' the emotional undercurrent of the person's life. It is only when a meaningful connection is formed with another who listens and can 'hear' the felt experience that new meaning can be co-created and a more reality-based perspective can be constructed.

Having an honest conversation with my partner early on gave us both the chance to explore each other's responses to the internal chaos resulting from the high levels of anxiety and uncertainty that we were sharing. Perhaps reflecting a way of being which might be common in most couples, we realised that fear and hope were split between us, leaving us each to carry the opposite feeling. Looking back, I see how this may have unconsciously created a form of respite for us both, each of us knowing that the other was able to stay in touch with the feeling that we ourselves could not bear. Hope, which my partner found difficult to hold onto, can be unbearable too. Together, we managed to create a more realistic and whole picture, each of us balancing the other, keeping us from spinning out of control.

But what of my seven-year-old daughter, Carmen? Where might her mind take her? What lies in the unconscious of a child who is facing a life-threatening illness? What phantasies arise from the fear of separation and the disconnection from the mother, the source of life and nourishment? What does a child imagine, facing the unknown alone? What sense might be made of the loss not only of life, but of the possible future self they may have become? These kinds of questions, about which we can only speculate, were very much alive for me during the whole period spanning Carmen's hospitalisation and follow-up treatment. However, as I was to discover, my daughter had her own, and very different, experience.

The figure of Peter Pan welcomes every child at the entrance to London's Great Ormond Street Hospital (GOSH), one of the world's leading children's hospitals. J.M. Barrie donated the rights from his book to GOSH and Parliament made an exemption to the law to ensure this copyright never expires. It is thought that Barrie may have based the character of Peter Pan on his older brother, David, who died in an ice-skating accident the day before his 14th birthday. His mother and J.M. Barrie himself saw David as 'forever a boy'.

This story of a child who refuses to grow up and lives through wonderful adventures in Neverland grew in meaning for me during the time I spent in GOSH. Staying in the hospital was presented to children as a magical ride where opportunities for fun are constantly on offer and can be engaged in anytime when not going through an intervention. Magicians, singers, playful nurses, and therapists can be found on the wards alongside the doctors and other medical staff. This creates an extreme, almost surreal, contrast between an abundance of pleasure and the harsh reality of serious illness and even death, along with an intensity of feeling. Each child and parent can find themselves on a quest of discovery where challenges of every kind are a constant companion, all contributing to the unfolding of their own, still to be written, tale.

Peter Pan is the friend whose self-appointed role is to take care of the lost children. Wendy and her brothers are allowed to visit the mythical island of Neverland but after facing both delight and danger, choose to go back to the safety of their mother and resume the process of growing up. The resonances of this story shine with meaning for every child; in the context of GOSH, children are unconsciously presented with what could be internalised by them as the possibility of a good ending where recovery may be represented by the returning to the safety of their bond with their mother. Conversely, death might symbolise never growing up and staying in the fun of Neverland forever. In each case, children win out.

Sourkes describes the child's awareness of the life-threatening implications of their disease as being on a continuum. At one end, the child acknowledges being 'very sick' but with no prognostic statement referring to life or death. In the middle, awareness of the disease arouses in the child an uncertainty about living, but without a focus on death. At the other extreme, the child is aware that he or she could die of the illness. Awareness can be gleaned from many sources, such as the child's age, their growing understanding of the illness, the speed at which their medical treatment is set into motion, the emotions of family or caregivers and encounters with other patients.

The urgency surrounding my daughter Carmen's treatment began with her diagnosis and continued through the nine-month period to follow which included surgery, intense radiotherapy and chemotherapy. All of this was an evident sign of the severity of her illness, as was the immediate response of our large extended families who were in daily contact throughout the long months of treatment, offering unconditional support and nurturing which served as an invaluable source of containment. If there was an awareness of the danger she was facing, Carmen didn't give into it, instead choosing to focus on living in the moment. She did not ask any further questions after the first one which was 'how did this get into my brain?', perhaps picking up on the doctor's inability to explain fully or satisfactorily where cancer cells come from.

When I returned to my school-based therapy work following Carmen's recovery, a young secondary school-aged client named Joyce was referred to me as she was awaiting brain surgery although not for the same reasons as my daughter. I discovered how differently children can respond to a serious health condition and the uncertainty that this brings in its wake. Unlike Carmen, Joyce had many questions about the complicated operation she was soon to undergo and her mother was unsure about how to respond. The impact of 'telling' versus 'not telling' the child the extent of their illness has received much attention over the years. In the past the stance taken was not to share the diagnosis with the child in an attempt to shield them from anxiety and fear. However, in the last two decades, there has been a shift towards more honest communication. Usually the approach is to limit the initial information provided while offering the child an open invitation to ask for more as and when they wish to. This creates a safety valve, allowing the child to take the lead on how much they want, or need, to know and when.

I used a similar strategy in supporting Joyce and her mother. To help contain their anxieties and to give Joyce the chance to voice her concerns, I suggested she write down on slips of paper all her worries and questions around her upcoming surgery and put them into a specially created 'worry box'. Joyce's mother and I agreed to set a specific time each week when they would take out the slips and go through them together. I arranged to ring on the same day to speak to them both. This quickly brought down their anxiety levels and improved their capacity to cope with the uncertainty of their situation. Taking control of their thoughts was helped by knowing there was a dedicated space and time to focus on them, leaving their minds less preoccupied with worry the rest of the time.

Listening closely to a child and being honest with them creates an atmosphere of trust. As the treatment progresses the child's feelings may change, so it is important to stay attuned to what can be a fluctuating need for information (Sourke, 1995). Returning to my daughter's experience, Carmen occupied her days in the hospital with endless hours of drawing, entertaining staff and other adults with jokes, and facing her everyday challenges with a mostly positive attitude. In short, she was a model of resilience. I felt I couldn't be anything less than that, and although this helped me to rise above my conscious fears, surrendering to her wise focus on the present and spending precious time with her, it was at times hard to hold my (and most likely her) unconscious anxieties at bay. In such situations, the child's unarticulated feelings can be projected into the mother, who can act as a container for them. Carmen's passion for drawing and creating stories didn't diminish during her treatment, providing her with an additional channel for her unconscious expression. The mother in me couldn't help but observe her through the eyes of the therapist I also was. Looking at her pictures and reading her stories, it was impossible not to see representations of what Carmen was facing but I also saw hope, leaving me feeling touched by their significance.

Another client of mine, Esther, a slightly older secondary school student with some special needs, also used art-making to good effect in her sessions with me. Before I began with her, I was told by her Head of Year that she had been hospitalised on many occasions since she was a baby due to kidney failure and had already undergone an unsuccessful kidney transplant. After a lifelong experience of doctors and hospital interventions, Esther was reluctant to take up any professional support and had consistently refused to see a therapist to help her make sense of and manage her understandable angry outbursts and communication difficulties with her family and friends. Esther was going to have to face another transplant operation soon. Given the high anxiety and non-compliance she displayed, it was considered a priority to help her to regulate her emotions and to feel she had some agency over the upcoming life-saving intervention.

Fortunately, I discovered from one of her teachers that Esther had a passion for puppet making and drama, interests that I shared. I was able to use this to encourage her to come to the therapy room for our first session. From my conversations with the school and with Esther's mother, I anticipated that our relationship might well be difficult to establish at least at first, due to her past experiences with health professionals. One of the most disturbing aspects of illness is the sense that we are powerless over our lives, our bodies, and even our minds at times. For a child who has literally been under the caring, although also frightening, hands of doctors, puppets can offer a perfect inversion of roles that go some way towards restoring the child's sense of control. Over the years I have been building up a collection of hand-made puppets, and I invited Esther to help me repair and restore some of my older ones. We quickly became the equivalent of doctors and nurses on 'operation duty'. I soon learned that any reference to her own hospital life, however oblique, was responded to with rage and anxiety which Esther didn't seem to have the inner resources to manage. At this stage in the therapy, our work with the puppets was particularly potent and touching, enabling us to symbolically play out many different scenarios.

Over time, as the date of the surgery grew closer, my conversations with Esther's mother rarely moved off the topic of practical arrangements and what might be involved in the treatment plan. Although Esther and I were still not speaking openly about the operation, reality began to make itself felt and Esther's defences were triggered. Working with the puppets had provided a medium through which Esther could metaphorically express a range of feelings and fantasies, perhaps rooted in non-verbal early life trauma. However, as the operation drew nearer, a conscious awareness of what was coming broke through. Esther began to use her therapy time with me to rage about 'having to attend', but without appearing able to leave the room or to consider pausing our sessions. My role throughout this period was to contain her raw feelings of anger, fear and powerlessness while verbalising how difficult it can be if we feel we've lost control of our lives, something I knew all too well due to my own unconscious responses when my life spun off track.

When the time came for Esther's operation, our relationship had deepened due to what we'd been through and the connection I'd built with her as well as with her mother and the hospital-based professionals who wanted me to prepare Esther for the coming hospital admission. We had survived much together, and in the process, made it possible for Esther to get through her hospital stay with less distress than had been anticipated.

At various stages throughout my work with Esther, I wondered whether to share with Esther's mother aspects of my own experience, but it seemed enough to be able to understand what she was going through and make use of what

I had learned from my time with my daughter. Just as therapy incorporates a 'felt experience' with conscious and unconscious identifications moving back and forth, so too did this feature in my regular contact with Esther's mother. We often spoke of practicalities including what was happening next on Esther's treatment plan. My role was a dual one: I was holding both the unconscious matrix and also containing the weight of the very conscious worries around the hospital stay that Esther's mother herself had to carry. Details emerged which were not dissimilar to what I had gone through with Carmen, even including the possibility of Esther being allocated to the same ward Carmen had been on. I wondered at times if Esther's mother would notice that I seemed very familiar with hospital procedures and with the experience of caring for a seriously ill child, hinting at what I, too, had been through. However, Esther's mother did not allude to this at any point and I intuitively understood that it was necessary to preserve the asymmetry of our relationship. Even though our experiences mirrored each other's so clearly, I instinctively grasped that what Esther and her mother needed from me was akin to taking up the role of a 'good enough parent' who would not be overwhelmed by unconscious fears or become defensively focused on trying to 'make things better'.

Perhaps the time will come when sharing my own experience may have a role to play in the therapeutic process. Tanner (2020) states that mutuality and asymmetry must be calibrated in line with the patient's individual needs which are variable and change over the course of treatment (Kuchuck, 2021). Mapping my struggles the way that I am doing could be a useful first step and, should I find myself with a similar client again, the viability of shifting to a more mutual relationship with the child and parent at some point during the therapy, could be developed, possibly in the final phase of the work. It could be that this would make it possible for the parent and even the child (depending on their age) to better arrive at an internal understanding that the seemingly 'un-survivable' can be lived through.

Interestingly, at the same time as seeing Esther, I was working at a different school with another mother and her son, Imran, who was younger than both Esther and Joyce. Like them, he was also awaiting brain surgery. In all these instances, following the medical processes step by step with the parent and the child meant reactivating some of my own wounds. This was brought home to me when I rang Imran's mother to find out how his surgery had gone. As Imran was closest to the age my daughter had been when she was hospitalised, I felt most acutely a familiar mix of the kind of impatience and dread I'd had when ringing to learn the outcome of Carmen's final MRI tests.

My reawakened emotions triggered by personal experiences with my daughter's illness added a unique depth to the therapeutic connection with all four of these children and their mothers. The more we are able to embrace our own woundedness, the less we need to protect our clients from the pain of feeling theirs. This in turn opens up the possibility of recognising the paradox at the heart of our profession: that the healing of the client's wounding in therapy is inseparable from the enactment of that wounding via the therapeutic relationship and through the therapist. Therefore, in order to access the transformative possibilities of therapy, I needed to be capable of allowing this enactment of the wounding to take place; that is to say, I had to be able to allow myself to become – and to be experienced – not only as the wounded, but also as the wounding healer.

In *How to Survive as a Psychotherapist* (2021), Nina Coltart describes something like this as 'learning to deploy two paradoxically contrasting states of being at one and the same time' (45: Ibid.). She says that it is only because we can be anxious (or afraid or any other difficult emotion) without trying to defend against that feeling or get away from it, that we can constructively approach another's anxiety (or other disturbing feelings). Although as therapists we have all gone through our own psychotherapy, Coltart goes on to say that this "does not take away our capacity for anxiety, depression and confusion, but we have learned different ways of handling these, new ways of 'staying with it', whatever 'it' is" (Ibid.). When working with a client who is going through something so emotionally charged which we, too, have experienced, it is the 'staying with it' which shows the client that the feelings aroused, no matter how frightening, are, in fact, survivable.

When Carmen's treatment ended successfully, which we marked with joyous celebrations, we couldn't wait to start a new chapter. Gratitude and relief filled our lives for some time. It was not until some months later that my anxiety began to creep back in. As Carmen adjusted to school life, I found myself reacting with disproportionate worry about any physical symptoms she manifested. It was my professional curiosity that led me to a therapeutic workshop designed to release creative blocks. The workshop themes centred around ritual, art and therapy and the series was led by a drama therapist. The idea was to create the story of a fictitious character (acknowledging it was a version of oneself) who undertakes a journey to face their greatest fear, dying after the first attempt but finding the strength to come back and defeat it. Part of the process was to mark each stage with a self-created ritual to acknowledge and celebrate our own symbolic death, discovery, rebirth, and victory over our fears. This work helped me make sense of what I had experienced living through Carmen's illness and to get in touch with the feelings that had been left unprocessed. I realised that I had to allow myself to become the frightened victim, the lost soul, the discoverer, and finally the hero of my own story in order to own it and feel some control over it.

Throughout my work as a therapist, most notably with Joyce, Esther, Imran and Akyra the theme of self-disclosure has moved in and out of the frame. To date, I have not made any explicit reference to my own experience either with a client or with their parent or carer. However, questions about whether, and if so when, a therapist's open disclosures might be warranted, have been around in the background. This became even more relevant when my daughter, after years of working collaboratively with a theatre maker who had experienced cancer himself, released an online interactive story to convey her own journey through her illness, the challenges she faced and the lessons she could extract from it (https://originofcarmenpower.co.uk). I felt divided about whether to share this online film with the children I worked with and/or their parents, thinking that it could be a great source of positivity and reassurance, but mindful of the impact that this could have on the therapeutic process. As Kuchuck (2021) states "the mere act of contemplating whether or not to make a disclosure – whether it be biographical, sharing of an affect, thought or insight of any kind – can become part of a therapeutic action (in a manner that differs from an actual explicit disclosure)". Although I was clear about the need to keep my personal life outside of the therapy, witnessing children and their mothers going through such similar journeys to mine made me consider disclosing some aspects of my own experience and questioning if, or how, this could be useful to my clients.

Even if I refrained from revealing her relationship to me, showing the film of my daughter's story to my clients with its upbeat message and happy ending could have given them a dose of hope but might have been at the cost of staying with the intensely uncomfortable fear and uncertainty that I knew so well. I was also aware of the consequences seeing the film might have on the unconscious dynamics at play. Transferential feelings of envy could be stirred if their treatment didn't have a similarly positive outcome and if no film was made of *them*. As it turned out, this very personal piece, only relatively recently completed by my daughter, was to be shown to the patients at the hospital where two of my clients received their treatment. Therefore, there was a slim possibility that they would have seen it and maybe even connected it to me. It is here that the wounded healer archetype reminds me how outdated the old model of the therapist as 'fully analysed' has become in contrast to a more relevant emphasis on the notion of embracing our own vulnerabilities as an inescapable and useful aspect of what we bring to the therapeutic relationship. As Kuchuck (2021) reflects, the personal and the technical are inseparable (Frank, 2005) and often our clearest thinking comes from the third space that arises as a result of the dialectic between the theoretical and the affective (Kuchuck, 2021). Therapy is very much a 'live' process which both shapes and is moulded by the unconscious communications and psychic material of both therapist and client.

Writing this chapter has put me back in touch with aspects of my history as well as my emotional responses to my work. It has been written in the hope that my story will enrich thinking more generally about how we work with parents and children facing a life-threatening illness as well as prompt further enquiry and research into the subject of personal disclosure.

References

Cain, N.R. (2000), Psychotherapist with Personal Histories of Psychiatric Hospitalisation: Countertransference in Wounded Healers. *Psychiatric Rehabilitation Journal*, 24(1), 22–28.

Coltart, N. (1993, Sheldon Press; Reissued 2021), *How to Survive as a Psychotherapist*, Phoenix Books, Bicester Oxfordshire.

Frank, K.A. (2005), *Towards Conceptualising the Real Relationship in Therapeutic Action: Beyond the Real Relationship, Psychoanalytic Perspectives*, Taylor and Francis (Online).

Kuchuk, S. (2021), *The Relational Revolution*, Confer Books, London.

Sourkes, B.M. (1986), *Armfuls of Time: The Psychological Experience of the Child with a Life-Threatening Illness*, Routledge, London and New York.

Tanner, J.G. (2020), Symmetry and Mutuality in the Imaginary: Analyzing the (Lack of) Structure. *Psychoanalytic Psychology*, 37(2), 158–164.

Epilogue

Lyn French

'Education, education, education' was the Labour government's defining mantra when it swept to power in 1997, the same year **A Space for creative learning and support** opened. It was originally set up as a research and development project by the Glass-House Trust (a Sainsbury Family Charitable Trust) in collaboration with the Social Science Research Unit at the Institute of Education, University of London, and the London Borough of Hackney's education department. The overarching aim was to provide school-based multi-partnered services in and out of curriculum time to meet the holistic needs of children and young people. It was a heady time when change for the better was in the air.

Over its 25-plus year history, A Space has gone through many different phases in its evolution leading to what it is today: a psychotherapy service working with children and young people in East London and seeing staff for counselling or supervision. Of our original collaborators working with us in the early days, we have retained a partnership with the **Institute of International Visual Arts (Iniva)** based at Chelsea College, University of the Arts. With the Stuart Hall Library acting as its creative hub, Iniva works with artists, curators, researchers, and cultural producers to engage in discourse and debate on issues reflecting the politics of race, class and gender. Focusing on themes relating to difference and diversity, A Space and Iniva continue to co-publish emotional learning resources and deliver a small, targeted programme of artist and therapist-led psycho-educational projects.

Reflecting our roots in research and development, we use our current therapy provision as a form of action research, adapting and refining our ways of working in response to what we discover along the way and sharing this across the psychotherapy community through publishing books, supervising non-A Space therapists, and developing resources. *Bringing our Histories into School-based Therapy* is our third and latest endeavour, intended to contribute to on-going thinking about how we can apply what we've learned from our personal experiences – knowledge often hard won – to our work with our young clients.

In keeping with the spirit of this book, I, too, will look beneath the surface and share some thoughts on the evolution of A Space from a more personal perspective. We know from the Tavistock's consultations with organisations that

DOI: 10.4324/9781003270447-18

wherever we go, we bring ourselves (Obholzer 2021; Cardona 2020; Obholzer and Zagier Roberts 2019; Hinshelwood 2000). Our unconscious agendas shape the career choices we make and have the potential to propel us forward as well as to distort, stall, or derail our efforts, sometimes in equal measure. Reflecting on my initial interest in the A Space project, I can see how themes that had pre-occupied me in my own therapy at that time played a part. Some years before, my mother had passed away from breast cancer which had rapidly metasta-sised. At the time of her death, I had only recently returned to London after completing a Fine Art degree in Canada and further studies. The year after she died, I trained in art psychotherapy which took me into adult psychiatry in the NHS. I then began the Tavistock MA in Observational Studies which focuses on infant, child, and adolescent development explored from a psychoanalytic perspective – ostensibly the first step towards taking on a second psychotherapy training. Possibly more accurately, it represented an attempt to reconnect with my mother via an identification with her own unrealised ambition to work with children and families either in social care or in some therapeutic capacity which was stalled when we moved from Canada to London because of my father's job. What was to be a two-year stay in the UK evolved into a permanent re-location and the studies she had embarked on were left behind.

By moving from a job in adult psychiatric services to working at what became known as A Space, I was, on one level, 'picking up the baton' and carrying on where my mother had left off, both linking with her in mind as well as making reparation for those aspects of our relationship which had been left unresolved at the time of her death – all part of the mourning process. Needless to say, other ways of looking at my professional trajectory could be put forward and different interpretations made. There will always be a web of internal and external realities and influences motivating our choices – some contradictory, others synchronous – not all of which can be identified. As many of this book's chapter authors have noted, our relationship with our personal histories is dynamic, complex, and ever-evolving; there is no one 'true' version of our story or a single defining interpreta-tion to settle on, much as we might be tempted to neatly package it up.

Returning to that long ago date in September 1997, I can still vividly re-call the potent mix of excitement and trepidation I felt when I was readying myself to take up a senior project development officer's role on the original A Space team under the lead of the then-Director, Keith Jennings. Looking back evokes memories of what psychotherapist Ricky Emanuel (2000) describes as 'the uncertainty cloud' that descends whenever we engage in something new which has significance for us. This 'cloud' contains all our doubts, rational and otherwise, about our abilities, including how we imagine others might see us as well as fears that we might fail to meet the expectations of those whose positive regard we most value. Among these figures are any 'good objects', past or pres-ent, who occupy an important place in our internal world.

In any workplace, there is always what Francesca Cardona (2021) describes as a 'shadow anxiety' in the background linked to the fear of failing and what this means to each member of the team or organisation. Starting a service from scratch brings with it an expectation, real or otherwise, of making it a success. This was especially so at A Space with the researchers, funder and steering group all looking on. Being the recipient of the other's gaze is always a potent experience. Regardless of the reality, we can read it as benign or persecutory, admiring or shaming. In all likelihood my pendulum swings back and forth between these poles reflected what others on the team felt too.

Much that is written about by those who analyse work dynamics also applied at A Space back in the beginning. With all team members being new to their post, and specialisms overlapping in places, collaboration had to be managed so it didn't tip into unhelpful rivalry and competition, easier at some points than others. Staying in touch with reality was painful at times, too. In a chapter entitled 'On Beginnings' in *Workplace Intelligence: Unconscious Forces and how to Manage Them*, Anton Obholzer (2021) suggests that focusing only on the hopes or, conversely, the fears makes for a disjointed approach, "giving the message that the other half of the emotional equation, whether hopeful or hopeless, cannot be thought about". He goes on to say: "In reality, there are no 'win/win situations', popular though this concept might be" (Ibid.:13). Even so, there is no denying that the idea of a win/win is a seductive one, sidestepping as it does the internal effort required to deal with complexities, ambiguities and negatives of any kind including our own ambivalence about engaging in this form of psychological work. On the surface, A Space had all the hallmarks of a win/win – the right political context, the funding opportunities, the innovative spirit – making it tempting to construct a 'creation story' that focuses solely on the successes, of which there were many.

However, we probably all felt from the start the discomfort of being based in Kingsland Secondary, known locally in Hackney as a 'failing school', one that was destined to be closed and torn down to become one of the then-Labour government's new academies. We witnessed the painful reality: students (including, of course, those we worked with) slowly disappearing as they were transferred in batches to other local schools which were instructed by the government to make room for them, relegating them to the dubious position of 'educational refugees'.

Much as we hoped that A Space might successfully navigate the developmental pathway through conception, birth and its 'growing up' years to become an established service, it was never a given. As illustrated in different ways in each of the chapters in this book, all aspects of our world are heavily inflected by the 'knowns' and 'unknowns' as well as the spin we put on them, consciously or otherwise. Organisations are no different, for what are they, other than a collection of individuals, each with their story to tell? The fact that the A Space provision continues to be a viable service could be said to be, in part, the result of a dovetailing of the internal motivations of those who have contributed over the years with various external realities including shifts in government priorities, related policy changes, and a growing demand for school-based mental health provision.

Other factors are of equal – and significant – importance such as the continuity provided by the involvement of the Steering Group Chair Nicola Baboneau from the start as well as the ongoing support of the founder, Alex Sainsbury and his Trust, the Glass-House and a key Trustee, Elinor Jansz. As organisational consultants note, effective leadership primarily rests on identifying, containing, and interpreting anxiety and helping team members in facing it, something that is most attainable if there is a 'secure base' in the background (Cardona 2021). In the current work environment which increasingly requires therapy organisations to be responsive to fast-moving changes with insecure or time-limited funding often the norm, A Space has benefited from relative security. This has made it possible to provide a professional home for many therapists and the not-to-be-taken-for-granted chance to reflect and innovate, adapting our practice and sharing our learning.

One could say that, at least for the present and hopefully the future too, we have fulfilled what, from the start, has been central to our primary purpose: creating *a space* in the minds of educationalists and government policy makers for more relational-based thinking. This includes providing the kind of opportunities A Space offered in its first phase of development for emotional learning via arts, sports and cultural initiatives through to ensuring that in-school therapy and staff counselling and supervision remain on the agenda. Whether A Space continues longer term in its current form or not, the countless therapists who have been part of our service at one time or another have made an invaluable contribution to 'birthing' and 'keeping alive' the idea that we can all benefit from *a space* to talk, feel, reflect, process, play, and imagine. As Adam Phillips so poignantly put it in an interview with Ed Corrigan,

> I think the thing Winnicott said is right, that there's no such thing as a separation, there's only the fantasy of separation. And people that we've been really moved by and loved or been affected by or whatever, they stay with us. And it doesn't mean there's no loss in life or anything like that. I just mean relationships go on in different forms, they evolve ….
>
> (Phillips 2019:71)

References

Cardona, F. (2020) *Work Matters: Consulting to Leaders and Organisations in the Tavistock Tradition*. London: Routledge.

Hinshelwood, R.D. (2000) *Observing Organisations: Anxiety, Defence and Culture in Healthcare*. London: Routledge.

Obholzer, A. (2021) *Workplace Intelligence: Unconscious Forces and How to Manage Them*. London: Routledge.

Obholzer, A., Zagier Roberts, V. eds (1994) *The Unconscious at Work: Individual and Organizational Stress in the Human Services*. London: Routledge.

Obholzer, A., Zagier Roberts, V. eds (2019) *The Unconscious at Work: A Tavistock Approach to Makings Sense of Organizational Life*. London: Routledge.

Phillips, A. (2019) *The Cure for Psychoanalysis*. London: Confer Books.

Index